Chair Yoga for Seniors

The Ultimate Illustrated Guide
to Enhance Strength, Balance, and Mobility
with 15-Minute Daily Low-Impact
Seated Exercises | Suitable for All Skill Levels

Written by:

Peggy Mitchell

Copyright © 2024
All rights reserved.

Table of Contents

Chapter 1: Introduction to Chair Yoga for Seniors 1

Welcome to Chair Yoga for Seniors 1
Understanding the Benefits of Chair Yoga 2
Addressing Common Misconceptions About Yoga for Seniors 4
Empowering Self-Assessment for Chair Yoga 6
The Chair Yoga Revolution: What Sets This Book Apart 8

Chapter 2: Preparing for Chair Yoga Practice 9

Setting Goals and Establishing Realistic Expectations for Chair Yoga 10
Selecting the Ideal Chair for Chair Yoga: A Journey of Comfort and Safety 11
Creating the Perfect Space for Chair Yoga: A Haven of Serenity and Safety 13

Chapter 3: The 5 Key Benefits of Chair Yoga for Mental Well-Being and Mindfulness 15

1. Harmonizing Mind and Body 16
2. Improving Cognitive Clarity and Emotional Wellness 17
3. Adopting a Holistic Path to Physical, Mental, and Spiritual Wellness 19
4. Harnessing the Transformative Power of Chair Yoga 20
5. Incorporating Meditation and Mindfulness into Practice 21

Practical Applications and Exercises 23

Chapter 4: The Power of Yoga Mudras 29

Introducing to Yoga Mudras and Their Benefits 29
Incorporating Mudras Into Your Chair Yoga Practice: A Holistic Approach 30
In the Journey of Mudras: Ten Timeless Gestures in Chair Yoga 33

Chapter 5: Gentle Warm-Up and Cooldown 43

The Art of Warming Up 43
Warm Up Practices 44

The Grace of Cooling Down 47

Cooldown Practices *48*

Chapter 6: Seated Poses for Strength, Flexibility, and Balance 52

A Variety of Seated Yoga Poses 52

The Benefits of Structured Yoga Routines 52

Routine 1 .... *54*

Routine 2 .... *68*

Routine 3 .... *82*

Developing Core Strength and Flexibility 96

Chapter 7: Chair Yoga for Upper and Lower Body Health 101

Targeting Neck, Shoulder, and Arm Strength 101

Routine 1: Alleviating Tension and Pain in the Upper Body *103*

Routine 2: Exercises for Enhanced Posture *120*

Enhancing Leg Strength and Mobility 136

Routine 1: Preventing Falls and Improving Balance *138*

Routine 2: Targeted Exercises for Leg and Hip Wellness *154*

Chapter 8: Chair Yoga Regimens: Tailored for Results 170

15-Day Chair Yoga Journey: Training and Progress Tracking 170

15-Day Chair Yoga Training: Progress Monitoring Tools 171

Days 1 to 5: Laying Down the Foundations *174*

Tailored Checklist Routine for Days 15 .... *180*

Days 6 to 10: Boosting Strength in Upper and Lower Body *181*

Tailored Checklist Routine for Days 6 to 10 .... *188*

Days 11 to 15: The Whole Package *190*

Tailored Checklist Routine for Days 11 to 15 .... *198*

Conclusion 199

Chair Yoga: A Practice for a Lifetime 199

Glossary 201
　Introduction 201
　How to Use This Glossary 201

Acknowledgments

This book is presented below with the utmost commitment to accuracy and reliability in providing information. However, it's important to understand that purchasing this book implies an acknowledgment that neither the publisher nor the author of this book claim expertise in the topics discussed. Any recommendations or suggestions presented here are intended for entertainment purposes only. For any professional guidance or actions related to the content herein, it is advisable to consult with qualified experts.

This declaration is recognized as fair and valid by both, the American Bar Association and the Committee of Publishers Association, and it holds legal validity throughout the United States.

Furthermore, any form of transmission, duplication, or reproduction of the following work, including specific information, is considered illegal, whether conducted electronically or in print. This prohibition extends to creating secondary or tertiary copies of the work or recorded versions and is permissible only with the express written consent of the Publisher. All additional rights are reserved.

The information presented in the following pages is generally considered a truthful and accurate account of facts. Consequently, any actions taken by the reader based on this information are solely their responsibility. Under no circumstances can the publisher or the original author of this work be held liable for any difficulties or damages that may arise as a result of applying the information described herein.

Moreover, the information provided in the following pages is intended solely for informational purposes and should be regarded as such. It is presented without guarantee of its long-term validity or immediate relevance. Mention of trademarks is not done with written consent and should not be construed as an endorsement from the trademark holder.

Chapter 1: Introduction to Chair Yoga for Seniors

Welcome to Chair Yoga for Seniors

In our ever-evolving journey of life, as we advance in age, the quest for well-being takes on new dimensions. Traditional exercises, once a breeze, may now present daunting challenges. But fear not, for not every path to wellness demands the sprightliness of youth. Enter the realm of Chair Yoga, a hidden gem for those gracefully embracing their later years, revealed in the pages of *Chair Yoga for Seniors*.

This book is a treasure trove that interweaves physical rejuvenation with mental and spiritual nourishment. Each movement, every mindful breath, and all moments of tranquility are meticulously curated to not only enhance physical agility and strength but also to enrich mental clarity and instill a sense of calm.

Designed for those gracefully navigating the later chapters of life, our approach in *Chair Yoga for Seniors* is one of gentle encouragement and holistic nurturing. Prepare to embark on a journey of rediscovery, to find balance, and to embrace harmony at any age.

So, settle in your chair and begin this transformative adventure together. *Chair Yoga for Seniors* is your compass to a healthier, happier, and more harmonious existence, proving that true vitality knows no age.

Understanding the Benefits of Chair Yoga

Chair Yoga isn't merely another passing fitness trend; it signifies a genuine revolution in how seniors approach their health and wellbeing. In the following pages, we'll delve into the extraordinary and distinctive advantages that Chair Yoga brings. It's not just another exercise; it's a tailored practice designed specifically for seniors, with the potential to enrich physical, mental, and spiritual wellbeing. Let's uncover why Chair Yoga is an exceptional choice for seniors like yourself.

Universal Accessibility

Chair Yoga is rooted in the principle of accessibility. It extends a warm welcome to individuals of all ages and physical capabilities, offering a practice that can be customized to suit your unique requirements. Whether you're recuperating from an injury, navigating mobility constraints, or stepping into yoga for the first time, Chair Yoga invites you with open arms.

Enhanced Physical Wellbeing

Chair Yoga provides a gentle yet highly effective way to enhance physical health. It contributes to improved muscle strength, flexibility, coordination, and balance, vital attributes for preserving your independence and mobility as you age.

Elevated Mental Serenity

Beyond its physical facets, Chair Yoga exerts a profound influence on mental wellbeing. It fosters relaxation, mitigates stress, and sharpens mental acuity. Chair Yoga crafts a tranquil sanctuary for your thoughts through deliberate movements and mindful breathing.

Community and Camaraderie

Seniors sometimes grapple with social isolation, particularly when practicing Chair Yoga at home. Nevertheless, whether in person or through virtual classes, Chair Yoga sessions often nurture a sense of community and connection. Even in the comfort of your home, you can engage with kindred spirits who share your dedication to wellbeing. This sense of belonging to a broader community can bestow motivation, support, and a sense of togetherness upon your Chair Yoga journey.

Joint Friendly

Chair Yoga's standout feature is its low-impact nature. It bestows kindness upon your joints, rendering it an optimal choice for seniors contending with arthritis or joint discomfort. You can reap the rewards of exercise without subjecting your body to undue strain.

Mental Clarity and Tranquility

Beyond its physical aspects, Chair Yoga confers profound mental advantages. It advocates relaxation, stress reduction, and heightened mental lucidity. You'll discover an oasis of serenity for your mind by engaging in mindful movements and focused breathwork.

Tailored Solutions

This book refrains from adopting a one-size-fits-all approach. We comprehend that seniors confront unique challenges, such as persistent arthritis pain and the apprehension of falling. Chair Yoga offers tailored solutions and precise guidance to address these particular concerns. Importantly, you won't encounter standing poses in this book that might evoke the fear of falling, nor poses that necessitate lying on the floor—a predicament when it comes to rising back to your feet. Within these pages, you'll encounter solely seated poses, prioritizing your comfort and safety.

Prioritizing Safety

Safety is paramount in Chair Yoga. Utilizing a chair as a prop bestows added stability and support during your practice, reducing the risk of injuries.

Empowerment

Although you may harbor concerns regarding effectiveness and safety, your determination to enhance your well-being remains unwavering. Chair Yoga empowers you to seize control of your health and embark on a journey towards a more serene and pain-free life.

As you peruse this chapter further, you'll gain a deeper appreciation of these advantages and how Chair Yoga can wield a positive impact on your life. We will also address common misconceptions surrounding yoga for seniors and assist you in setting realistic objectives for your Chair Yoga practice.

So, let's immerse ourselves in exploring how Chair Yoga can chart your course to a healthier, happier, and more vibrant life, both physically and mentally.

Addressing Common Misconceptions About Yoga for Seniors

Yoga Is Just for the Young and Flexible

It's crucial to emphasize that yoga doesn't exclusively cater to the young and bendy crowd. Yoga spans a diverse spectrum of styles and complexities. Chair Yoga, in particular, has been meticulously crafted to extend its embrace to seniors, regardless of their mobility or flexibility levels. This approach revolves around a series of seated poses thoughtfully designed with gentleness and tailored to meet the unique needs of seniors. The objective isn't to pursue extreme flexibility or fancy postures; it's about discovering comfort and progressing at your own pace.

Yoga is Too Difficult for Seniors

The misconception that yoga is physically demanding often arises from certain vigorous yoga styles. However, Chair Yoga stands as a perfect choice for seniors precisely because of its gentle and low-impact nature. Chair Yoga places a premium on seniors' comfort and well-being, focusing on deliberate, unhurried movements, deep breathing, and relaxation. It's intentionally designed to be a soothing, stress-relieving practice, far removed from any strenuous or overwhelming expectations.

I'm Too Old to Start Yoga

Age should never serve as a deterrent to commencing a yoga practice. In reality, yoga can offer substantial benefits to seniors. As we age, preserving flexibility, balance, and mobility becomes increasingly pivotal for overall health and quality of life. Chair yoga provides a safe and effective way for seniors to work on these aspects of physical well-being, regardless of age or previous yoga experience. It's never too late to embark on a yoga journey that can enhance your health and vitality.

Yoga Is Only About Physical Poses

While physical postures represent a fundamental facet of yoga, they constitute just a fragment of the whole. Yoga adopts a holistic approach that encompasses not only physical health but also mental and emotional well-being. Chair Yoga places a strong emphasis on mindfulness, stress reduction, and relaxation techniques. Seniors who embrace Chair Yoga will encounter it as a gateway to mental clarity, emotional equilibrium, and inner serenity. It extends beyond mere physical movements to promote overall well-being.

I Have Physical Limitations, So I Can't Do Yoga

This misconception crumbles in the context of Chair Yoga. Chair Yoga stands out for its remarkable adaptability and accommodation of physical limitations. The chair itself functions as a sturdy prop that offers support during exercises. Seniors contending with various physical challenges, such as arthritis, restricted mobility, or balance issues, can partake in Chair Yoga exercises that are both secure and effective. Chair Yoga is intentionally designed to address these limitations, gently enhancing physical health in a controlled manner.

Yoga Is a Religion

Yoga undeniably has deep historical and philosophical roots and can be linked to spirituality for certain practitioners. Nevertheless, it's imperative to dispel the misconception that yoga itself is a religion. Yoga is, in fact, a multifaceted practice that can be approached in a secular and nonreligious manner. Chair Yoga, in particular, hones in on the physical and mental dimensions of the practice, rendering it accessible to individuals from diverse backgrounds and belief systems. It serves as a versatile practice that seamlessly integrates into one's daily routine without any religious connotations.

Empowering Self-Assessment for Chair Yoga

Embarking on your Chair Yoga journey begins with a powerful notion: the key to empowerment lies in recognizing your individual needs and capacities. In this section, we'll plunge into the art of self-assessment. By taking the reins of your self-assessment, you'll unlock valuable insights into your physical limitations and concerns, equipping you to customize your Chair Yoga practice to align with your unique requirements. This self-assessment process empowers you to engage in your practice securely and confidently, even in the absence of direct instructor guidance. Let's embark on a journey to explore how you can autonomously evaluate your physical readiness for Chair Yoga and tailor your practice accordingly.

Introspective Contemplation

Let's kickstart this journey with a moment of introspective contemplation. Find a comfortable seat, and pause to reflect on those areas of your body that may be harboring stiffness, discomfort, or a touch of resistance to flexibility.

Charting Your Health Odyssey

Now, let's dive into the pages of your medical history. Delve into any health adventures or surgical experiences you've had. Take note of any specific health considerations that may be on your radar.

The Limb Limbering Expedition

It's time to embark on an expedition to limber up those limbs! Gently take your joints through their full range of motion, exploring every direction. Offer your wrists, ankles, and neck a gentle twist, and allow your arms and legs to experience a benevolent stretch. Keep a watchful eye for any areas that may be holding onto stiffness or discomfort.

Balancing Act

How's your sense of balance, you daredevil? Attempt to rise from your chair without seeking assistance. If you find this endeavor a bit challenging, consider it a friendly nudge that your balance and stability might appreciate some attention.

Tools of the Trade

If you have some props on hand, such as cushions, blocks, or stretchy bands, introduce them to your practice. Discover how these props can extend a helpful hand—or should I say a helpful prop?

Steady as She Goes

When you're ready to immerse yourself in Chair Yoga, adopt a gentle and gradual approach. Opt for uncomplicated poses and movements that feel cozy, and as you find your rhythm, you can begin to add a bit of zest. There's no need to rush this journey!

The Body's Whisper

Here's a golden rule to heed. Your body holds the ultimate wisdom. If a particular movement or pose elicits any discomfort or that unmistakable "ouch," promptly ease off. Your body assumes the role of commander-in-chief in matters of safety.

Charting Progress

Within our guide's pages, we offer standardized methods for tracking your journey and precise metrics for designated routines. Secure a journal to document your expedition, recording any achievements in the realms of flexibility, balance, or strength. It serves as an unerring means to sustain your motivation without having to scour the internet or other sources.

Stay Informed

Remain well-versed in all matters of Chair Yoga. Seek out books, peruse articles, or indulge in videos that dissect the practice and its ingenious nuances.

And always remember, Chair Yoga is as adaptable as a chameleon. You have the power to finetune it to harmonize with your unique style and abilities. While having an instructor at your side is undoubtedly advantageous, these steps pave the path to self-assessment autonomy, ensuring that you can engage in your practice securely and confidently, at a pace that suits you best.

The Chair Yoga Revolution: What Sets This Book Apart

What sets *Chair Yoga for Seniors* apart is our unwavering dedication to providing a comprehensive approach to this practice. Beyond focusing solely on its physical aspects and the advantages it brings to the body, we place a special emphasis on mental health and holistic well-being.

Our holistic perspective on Chair Yoga embraces the profound connection between the body and mind, recognizing their intertwined influence. Each exercise, every breath, and each moment of mindfulness are carefully crafted not only to enhance muscle strength and flexibility but also to nurture mental clarity and foster relaxation. Through this practice, you'll find an opportunity to rediscover yourself, to attain equilibrium, and to embrace harmony.

Within the pages of this book, we will accompany you through exercises that extend beyond physical well-being, teaching you how to manage stress, alleviate anxiety, and cultivate serenity of the mind. This comprehensive approach is meticulously tailored to assist seniors in maintaining physical fitness and elevating the overall quality of their lives.

We extend an invitation to you to embark on a journey into the realm of Chair Yoga with an open heart and an open mind, prepared to explore the myriad benefits that this practice has to offer, not only to your body but also to your spirit and mind. Our aspiration is that this holistic perspective ignites within you a desire to pursue a state of enduring and all-encompassing well-being.

Chapter 2: Preparing for Chair Yoga Practice

Welcome to Chapter 2, your golden ticket into the enchanting world of Chair Yoga for seniors. Picture this chapter as your very own personal assistant, meticulously guiding you through the essential steps to comfortably embrace this wonderful form of exercise.

Imagine gearing up for a splendid garden party. You need the right spot, a magical setup, and a clear vision of your goals. But rest easy—no backbreaking gardening work here!

Let's start this journey with a sprinkle of enthusiasm, a dash of practical wisdom, and a hearty dose of humor. After all, every adventure should include a few chuckles, right?

As we delve into preparing for Chair Yoga, we'll keep things light and breezy—no need for heavy lifting here! From selecting the ideal chair that doesn't squeak with every move (we all know that one chair, don't we?) to creating a tranquil little nook for practice, we've got all the tips and tricks you need.

We'll also talk about setting realistic expectations. While aiming high is great, keeping our feet (or chairs, in this case) grounded is just as important. Think of Chair Yoga not as a race but more like a relaxing walk in the park—it's about enjoying each step of the journey, not just rushing to the finish line.

So, get ready to embark on this delightful adventure with open hearts and curious minds. In Chair Yoga, every small step is a triumph, and every stretch is a celebration of your amazing abilities. So, adjust your glasses (if you wear them), grab your favorite cushion, and let's get ready for a journey full of satisfying achievements and wonderful surprises!

Setting Goals and Establishing Realistic Expectations for Chair Yoga

Starting your Chair Yoga journey? Think of it as picking up a delightful new hobby. It's all about combining attainable goals and realistic expectations to create an experience that's both rewarding and wonderfully doable.

Crafting Personalized Goals

Chair Yoga is your new pet project. What's your aim? Seeking a tranquil mind, supple limbs, or maybe a softly strengthened core? Tailor those goals to your needs, be it easing discomfort, sharpening your mental edge, or simply snatching a serene slice out of a hectic day.

Embracing the Achievable

Chair Yoga isn't about racing to the finish line. It's more akin to a soothing amble through the park. Set those targets with your current abilities in mind. If touching the stars feels a bit much, aim for reachable feats—like nurturing your joints or savoring the serenity of a deep breath.

Mixing Goals With a Dash of Realism

It's all about balancing dreams with a healthy splash of reality. Some days, your Chair Yoga session might be about smooth, gentle movements. Other times, it might revolve around breathing and calmness. Keep your goals fluid, adapting to your everyday physical and emotional state.

Celebratory Tracking

Every small win in your Chair Yoga journey deserves a cheer. This book comes packed with specialized trackers, your cheerleaders, documenting every stride you make. Deeper stretches, and improved stability—every little enhancement counts and deserves a pat on the back.

Finding Harmony Between Ambitions and Acceptance

Blending your aspirations with a sprinkle of acceptance is vital. Chair Yoga is all about adaptability and kindness. Some poses might take a while to get the hang of, and that's perfectly okay. Respect your body's rhythm, as each session is a step toward your overall wellness.

Joy: Your Guiding Light

Let happiness be your compass in Chair Yoga. Each session is an opportunity to explore and celebrate your body's capabilities. As you align your goals with what's realistically achievable, your practice evolves into a journey of self-discovery and gentle progress.

By marrying goalsetting with realistic expectations in Chair Yoga, we strike a beautiful balance. This approach ensures your practice isn't just feasible but also a wellspring of joy and personal growth. Nurture your Chair Yoga path with patience and zest, and watch as it flourishes into a rewarding and enriching part of your life.

Selecting the Ideal Chair for Chair Yoga: A Journey of Comfort and Safety

Envision yourself as an explorer in quest of the perfect treasure: the chair that will transform your Chair Yoga into an unparalleled experience. Here are some invaluable tips for choosing your ideal travel companion:

- **Unwavering sturdiness:** Your dream chair should stand as a bastion of stability and safety. Ensure it can support your weight confidently without any hint of faltering. Test it: sit down and gently shift your weight around. Does it remain steadfast? Excellent!
- **Height matters, indeed!** The ideal chair allows you to plant your feet firmly on the ground, knees forming a graceful right angle. This detail not only enhances your dignified appearance but also aids in maintaining proper posture.
- **Comfort akin to an embrace:** The seat should be cozy, yet not a trap of excessive softness. Too plush? Farewell, stability. Too hard? Farewell, comfort. Strive for that perfect balance that cradles you without yielding.
- **Armrests? Better without:** A chair devoid of armrests grants you the freedom of a dancer. Your movements will be uninhibited and fluid. If you can't do without

them, ensure they don't hinder your graceful dance.

- **Back support, your trusty ally:** The chair should be a firm and loyal support for your back, preventing you from adopting camellike postures. Stay upright and proud, always!

- **No wheels or swivels, please:** Your chair should not become an amusement park ride. Stability is the keyword here. Wheels and swivel bases? They're better left in the office.

- **Practical and elegant materials:** Opt for materials that are easy to clean, like wood or metal, marrying elegance with practicality.

- **Size Does Matter:** The chair shouldn't be a throne for giants nor a perch for tots. Find one that fits you perfectly, allowing you to touch the ground with poise.

- **Simplicity for a delicate practice:** In Chair Yoga, less is indeed more. Adding a cushion or pillow can transform your practice into a true haven of wellbeing. Cushions and Pillows are faithful travel companions, they will softly support you, whether beneath your back, under your legs, or wherever you feel the need. A cushion on the seat? It's like sitting on a cloud.

- **Embrace comfort and safety:** Wrap yourself in the enchantment of Chair Yoga. With your trusty chair and a soft cushion, you'll create a corner of paradise. Here, it's not about heroic challenges but about enjoying a serene and healthy practice. Each session becomes a small ritual of peace and comfort.

- So, dear explorers, as you settle in for your next Chair Yoga session, let a simple cushion make the journey even sweeter and more enjoyable. Happy practicing, and may serenity always accompany you on your magical Chair Yoga journey!

Creating the Perfect Space for Chair Yoga: A Haven of Serenity and Safety

Embarking on your Chair Yoga journey doesn't require a vast or specialized space. The beauty of this practice lies in its ability to adapt to everyday environments. Here's how to create a safe and comfortable space for your Chair Yoga sessions, tailored to realistic home settings.

Choosing Your Space

Find a spot in your home where you feel calm and undisturbed. It could be a cozy corner of your living room, a quiet part of your bedroom, or even a peaceful nook in your study. The key is to find a location that exudes tranquility and invites relaxation. Ensure it's a space where you can close the door or ask for a bit of quiet time to practice without interruptions.

You don't need a lot of room—just enough to freely extend your arms and legs. Ideally, you should be able to stretch your arms out to the sides and overhead without touching anything. Also, there should be sufficient space in front of you to extend your legs and comfortably perform forward bends.

The Surface Matters

A flat and stable floor is crucial. Carpeted surfaces offer natural cushioning, perfect for comfort. If you have a hard floor, consider placing a nonslip yoga mat or a similar stable mat under your chair to prevent sliding and provide a bit of extra padding.

Lighting and Ambiance

Good lighting can enhance your practice. Natural light is ideal, so practicing near a window can be invigorating. However, ensure the light isn't too intense—soft, warm lighting can create a more relaxed atmosphere. You might also consider dimming the lights or using candles for early morning or evening sessions.

Minimizing Distractions

Strive to create a space free from distractions. Turn off or silence your phone, and if possible, inform your household members that it's your yoga time. A 'Do Not Disturb' sign can be a friendly reminder for others.

Personal Touches

Add personal elements that make the space feel special and conducive to relaxation. This could include a favorite plant, a small water fountain for soothing sounds, or even a cherished photo or artwork. The goal is to make this space uniquely yours.

Essential Accessories

Aside from your chair, keep a cushion or pillow handy for extra support. You might also want to have a blanket nearby for warmth on cooler days or added comfort in certain poses.

Keeping It Organized

After each session, take a moment to tidy up your space. Maintaining a neat and organized practice area invites positive energy and makes each session more inviting and free from distractions.

By thoughtfully setting up your Chair Yoga space, you create a personal sanctuary that supports your physical and mental wellbeing. It becomes a special place where you can explore the benefits of Chair Yoga, fostering a deeper connection with your practice. Remember, the goal is to create a space that feels safe, peaceful, and supportive, enriching your journey toward health and relaxation.

Chapter 3: The 5 Key Benefits of Chair Yoga for Mental Well-Being and Mindfulness

Welcome to Chapter 3, a chapter dedicated to delving into the less tangible yet equally essential aspects of Chair Yoga: mental well-being and mindfulness. As we journey through our later years, our quest evolves to encompass physical health and the nurturing of a serene mind and a spirit brimming with vitality. This chapter is an invitation into a world where the gentle flow of Chair Yoga meets the profound depths of mental tranquility.

Picture Chair Yoga as a serene river meandering through the landscape of our lives. On the one hand, our physical health is reinforced by every stretch and movement. On the opposite bank lies our mental state, a realm often left uncharted and undervalued, especially in our golden years. In this chapter, we bridge these two worlds, illustrating how Chair Yoga is not just about physical agility and strength but also about nurturing a peaceful mind and a resilient spirit.

Here, we'll explore the concept of the Mindbody connection, a cornerstone of Chair Yoga. This connection isn't merely a philosophical idea; it's a practical aspect of how our mental and physical health are deeply intertwined. When we lift an arm or gently twist in our chair, we move muscles and joints, influencing our thoughts, emotions, and overall mental health.

This chapter will guide you through cultivating a positive, growth-oriented mindset. Often, the challenges of aging cast shadows of doubt and limitation. However, Chair Yoga offers a different narrative, where each breath is an opportunity for growth, each movement a step toward positivity. We'll explore techniques and approaches that transform challenges into opportunities, fostering a mindset that embraces growth at every life stage.

Finally, we'll venture into the realms of meditation and mindfulness as integral parts of your Chair Yoga practice. Here, mindfulness isn't just a trendy buzzword; it's a tangible practice that enriches the Chair Yoga experience. We'll learn to incorporate mindful breathing and focused attention into our movements, transforming our practice into a form of moving meditation. This section is about bringing a quality of attentiveness to our practice, making each session a time of deep personal connection and tranquility.

As we journey through this chapter, remember that Chair Yoga is more than a physical practice. It's a path to a peaceful mind and a joyful spirit. It's about finding stillness in movement and clarity in moments of quiet. So, let's embark on this journey together, embracing the transformative power of Chair Yoga for mental health and mindfulness.

1. Harmonizing Mind and Body

At its core, Chair Yoga is not just a series of movements; it's a comprehensive experience that harmonizes the mind and body. This harmony is rooted in our body's biological responses, where physical actions significantly impact our mental wellness.

As we practice Chair Yoga, our bodies release endorphins, known as "happiness hormones," enhancing mood and reducing pain. These biochemical reactions are essential, especially in reducing stress hormones like cortisol, thereby promoting overall health. Additionally, Chair Yoga boosts neurotransmitters like serotonin and dopamine, which are crucial for emotional balance and happiness.

This practice is a virtuous cycle where each movement and breath nurtures both mental and physical well-being. It goes beyond physical exercise, serving as a holistic therapy that rejuvenates the mind and body. By embracing Chair Yoga, we nourish our entire being, understanding the profound impact of this mind-body connection.

Reducing Stress With Chair Yoga

Chair Yoga emerges as a tranquil oasis in our daily lives, countering stress effectively. It activates the parasympathetic nervous system, inducing relaxation and reducing physical signs of stress like high heart rate and blood pressure.

The thoughtful movements and deep breathing in Chair Yoga create a meditative state, providing physical calm and a mental break from stress. It's particularly effective for anxiety management, with deep breathing techniques sending calming signals to the brain and body.

Furthermore, Chair Yoga enhances concentration and mindfulness, allowing practitioners to immerse themselves in the present moment, away from daily stressors. This focus has a calming effect on the mind, making Chair Yoga a powerful tool for mental wellbeing. It's especially transformative for those in later years, offering serenity and balance during a phase of life often filled with challenges.

2. Improving Cognitive Clarity and Emotional Wellness

Chair Yoga, often celebrated for its physical benefits, is also a boon for mental and emotional strength. This gentle practice enhances cognitive clarity, bolstering concentration, memory, and mental agility, which is essential in the later chapters of life.

Mind Training

Chair Yoga is more than a physical routine; it's a mental workout. Each pose demands focus, sharpening the brain's ability to concentrate and enhancing cognitive functions. This mental discipline helps in strengthening concentration and attention skills.

Memory Boost

The practice stimulates both body and mind. Remembering sequences and focusing on breathwork utilizes both short-term and long-term memory, aiding in memory improvement essential for a fulfilling life in the senior years.

Present Moment Focus

Core to Chair Yoga is mindfulness. Concentrating on each movement and breath teaches practitioners to live in the now, enhancing everyday life and decision-making with clearer, more focused thinking.

Combatting Cognitive Decline

Studies suggest regular mental and physical activity can slow down age-related cognitive decline. Combining physical movement with mental concentration makes chair yoga a key tool for maintaining mental acuity.

Emotional Release Through Movement

Chair Yoga extends beyond physical benefits to emotional health. Specific poses, like forward bends, facilitate emotional release, allowing practitioners to let go of stress and reconnect with their inner selves.

Safe Emotional Exploration

In the comforting environment of Chair Yoga, individuals can confront and process emotions, especially those from challenging experiences. This safe exploration can lead to cathartic releases, empowering personal growth.

Building Emotional Resilience

Regular practice offers immediate emotional release and fosters long-term emotional resilience. By learning to release emotions healthily, practitioners can develop more effective coping strategies for future stress crisis.

In summary, Chair Yoga offers a holistic approach to wellness. It not only promotes physical strength and flexibility but also nurtures mental clarity and emotional well-being, making it an invaluable practice for those advancing in years.

3. Adopting a Holistic Path to Physical, Mental, and Spiritual Wellness

Chair Yoga is much more than a series of gentle movements; it's a holistic journey that harmoniously integrates the body, mind, and spirit. This practice offers profound benefits, from enhancing physical wellness to nurturing a deeper spiritual connection, particularly enriching for those embracing their later years.

At its core, Chair Yoga emphasizes body awareness. It encourages you to listen to your body attentively, recognizing subtle cues like muscle tension, breathing patterns, and emotional responses. This heightened awareness fosters a deeper understanding of how emotions manifest physically, such as stress-induced neck tension or anxiety in the chest. By being in tune with these bodily signals, you can more effectively manage stress, relax tense areas, and use breathwork to calm the mind.

Breathwork in Chair Yoga transcends its physical role, serving as a rhythmic guide to deeper mental focus and mindfulness. Concentrating on each breath's flow, practitioners can achieve a state of tranquility, distancing themselves from daily stressors and anxiety. This mindful breathing promotes relaxation and paves the way for a meditative state, enhancing mental clarity and emotional balance.

Moreover, Chair Yoga is a gateway to a profound spiritual journey. It encourages introspection, helping individuals explore their inner selves and discover insights about their life's purpose, joy, and serenity. This practice cultivates a sense of connectivity—with oneself, the surrounding world, and a higher spiritual realm for some. Integrating movement, meditation, and mindful breathing, Chair Yoga becomes a transformative experience, offering moments of deep relaxation that transcend the physical realm.

In summary, Chair Yoga is a nurturing practice that transcends mere physical exercise. It's a pathway to holistic wellness, enriching life with inner peace, deeper self-awareness, and a profound connection to the spiritual aspects of being. Whether it's through the mindful awareness of body and emotions, or the tranquil focus achieved through breathwork, Chair Yoga offers a comprehensive approach to wellness for people in their golden years and beyond.

4. Harnessing the Transformative Power of Chair Yoga

In Chair Yoga, the journey through physical postures and breathing exercises is far more than a path to physical wellness; it's a gateway to mental clarity, emotional balance, and, in many cases, spiritual exploration. This holistic approach makes chair yoga a powerful tool for harmonizing your inner world with the physical experience, leading to a richer and more balanced life.

On the Chair Yoga journey, each movement, each breath, becomes an opportunity for reflection, to listen to the silent dialogue between mind and body. It's an invitation to experience how calmness and mindfulness can infuse serenity into every aspect of life, turning it into an adventure enriched with profound awareness and joy.

For individuals, this practice becomes a voyage of rediscovery, where every small posture and every gentle movement becomes an act of self-love. Here, Chair Yoga transforms from mere physical activity to the poetry of movement, a silent language that tells stories of inner strength and tranquility.

So, dear readers, as you delve into the magical world of Chair Yoga, remember that each pose, each breath, is a step towards a more balanced and fulfilling life. It's a dance between body and mind that celebrates the beauty of every present moment, a hymn to life that resonates in the stillness of your sacred space.

On this journey, you will discover that Chair Yoga is not just a practice, but a way of life, a path leading to a deep wisdom and a peace deeply rooted in the heart. It's a discovery that each day can be lived with grace, with a clear mind and a heart full of peace.

5. Incorporating Meditation and Mindfulness into Practice

In the world of Chair Yoga, meditation emerges as a tranquil anchor, guiding participants toward a state of deep relaxation and enhanced awareness. It's not merely about sitting still; it's about nurturing an inner stillness that echoes through each movement.

Meditation in Chair Yoga can adopt various forms. Techniques such as focused breathwork, where each inhale and exhale is mindfully observed, or guided visualizations, which take participants on a mental journey, are widely embraced. Another approach involves the practice of mindful observation, providing a focal point for mental focus.

Meditation can be seamlessly integrated into Chair Yoga, whether before, during, or after the physical exercises. Beginning sessions with a short meditation can set a tone of mindfulness while concluding with meditation allows for the full absorption of the practice's benefits. Even brief meditative moments between poses can significantly enhance the overall experience.

Mindfulness in Chair Yoga is about fully embracing the present moment. It involves being keenly aware of each posture, the rhythm of the breath, the sensations in the body, and the emotions and thoughts that surface during the practice.

Encouraging participants to move with awareness, paying close attention to the transitions between poses and the alignment of their bodies, not only heightens the physical benefits of Chair Yoga but also fosters a deeper mental connection with the practice.

The mindfulness learned in the chair doesn't end with the session. Participants are encouraged to bring this heightened sense of awareness into their everyday activities, leading to a more mindful approach to life in general.

Through these practices, Chair Yoga transcends the realm of physical exercise, becoming a journey of personal growth and inner peace. It's a path that enhances physical wellness and enriches mental and emotional aspects, making every session a step toward a more mindful and fulfilling life.

Synergy Between Meditation and Mindfulness

In the world of Chair Yoga, the harmonious partnership between meditation and mindfulness creates a symphony of wellbeing. Meditation, with its tranquil depths, deepens the practice of mindfulness, making it more accessible and profound. Conversely, regular mindfulness practice paves the way for a smoother transition into a meditative state, like a gentle path leading into a serene forest.

Together, these practices form an all-encompassing approach that cares for the whole person. It's not just about physical health – though that's a significant part – but also nurturing the mental, emotional, and spiritual aspects. This holistic perspective is crucial for a truly enriching Chair Yoga experience, especially for those seeking more than just physical fitness from their practice.

Regular engagement in both meditation and mindfulness can lead to transformative changes. Imagine a world where stress and anxiety gently diminish, like clouds clearing after a storm, revealing a sky of clarity and calm. Cognitive functions, like memory and focus, improve as if the mind is being polished to a shine. Sleep deepens, each night becoming a rejuvenating journey. And overall, a profound sense of peace and wellbeing blossoms, much like a lotus flower emerging gracefully from the water.

In short, the synergy of meditation and mindfulness in Chair Yoga isn't just an addition to the practice; it's the heart of it. It's what changes each session from a series of movements and breaths into a journey of discovery, leading to a life lived with more depth, peace, and fulfillment.

Practical Applications and Exercises

In the gentle world of Chair Yoga, breath-focused practices become powerful tools for meditation and mindfulness. Let's explore some simple yet effective exercises:

Breath-Focused Practices

Simple exercises like observing the breath, counting breaths, or following the breath's journey through the body can be powerful meditation and mindfulness tools.

Exercise: Counted Breath

How to Do It: Settle comfortably in your chair, keeping your spine straight. Close your eyes and breathe normally. Start counting your breaths: inhale on count one, exhale on count two, and so forth, up to ten. Then start again at one. Continue for 5 minutes.

Benefits: This exercise sharpens focus and regulates breathing, promoting relaxation and easing stress. It's a perfect way to either start or wind down a Chair Yoga session.

Exercise: Alternate Nostril Breathing

How to Do It: Sit comfortably on your chair. Rest your left hand gently on your left knee. Place your right thumb over your right nostril and gently inhale through the left nostril. Then close your left nostril with your right finger, open your right nostril, and exhale slowly. Repeat this process, alternating nostrils with each breath. Continue for 5 minutes.

Benefits: This practice balances the left and right hemispheres of the brain, calms the mind, and improves focus and concentration.

Exercise: Ocean Breath

How to Do It: Sit comfortably in your chair, keeping your spine erect and shoulders relaxed. Begin by observing your natural breath without altering it. Gradually deepen your inhalation and exhalation, maintaining a smooth and steady rhythm. While breathing, subtly tighten the back of your throat to produce a gentle hissing noise akin to the sound of ocean waves during each inhalation and exhalation. It should be audible to you. Focus on the sound of your breath, allowing it to be slow and rhythmic. Continue this breathing technique for several minutes, feeling its calming effect on your mind and body.

Benefits: Ocean Breath is effective for calming the mind and warming the body. It aids in focusing the mind and is often used in yoga practices to enhance presence and awareness.

These breathing exercises are more than just routines; they are gateways to tranquility and heightened mindfulness, integral to the Chair Yoga journey. Through these practices, participants find physical ease and mental serenity, making each session a step towards a more mindful and enriched life.

Mindful Observation

In the enchanting realm of Chair Yoga, mindful observation emerges as a practice that teaches us to bring the same level of attention and mental presence into our everyday lives. Let's dive into some exercises that can help cultivate this important skill.

Exercise: Sensory Awareness

How to Do It: Sit quietly in your chair. Close your eyes and take a few deep breaths. Then, one by one, focus on each of your senses. What can you hear, smell, feel (like the chair against your skin), and taste? Spend a minute or two on each sense.

Benefits: This exercise heightens sensory awareness, rooting you in the present moment. It's excellent for developing mindfulness and can be particularly helpful during moments of anxiety or stress.

Exercise: Mindful Tea Drinking

How to Do It: Prepare a cup of tea and sit in your chair with the cup in your hands. Observe the steam rising, smell the aroma, feel the cup's warmth, and then slowly sip, paying attention to the taste and sensation as you drink. Engage in this activity mindfully, experiencing each aspect of drinking the tea.

Benefits: This practice increases mindfulness in everyday activities, helping to focus on the present and providing a sense of calm by engaging multiple senses.

Exercise: Color Spotting

How to Do It: Choose a color before you start. Throughout your day, whenever you notice something of that color, pause and observe it for a few seconds. Notice its shade, texture, and how it interacts with the surrounding space.

Benefits: This exercise enhances your present-moment awareness and helps you stay grounded. It also trains your mind to be more observant and attentive to your surroundings.

Through these exercises, Chair Yoga transforms into an experience that transcends the physical, becoming a pathway to enrich the mind and spirit. The practice of mindfulness teaches us to live each moment more fully, bringing to our daily lives a higher level of attention and tranquility, even in the little things.

Guided Imagery and Visualization

In the tranquil universe of Chair Yoga, guided imagery techniques emerge as precious allies, transporting participants to a state of deep relaxation and mental clarity. Here's how these techniques can be integrated into Chair Yoga practice, enriching the experience and bringing tangible benefits.

Exercise: Peaceful Garden Visualization

How to Do It: Sit comfortably and close your eyes. Take a few deep breaths to relax. Imagine yourself strolling through a magnificent, tranquil garden. Visualize the colors of the flowers, the sensation of a gentle breeze, and the sounds of birds. Mentally walk in this garden for 5 minutes, allowing yourself to be enveloped by a sense of peace and relaxation.

Benefits: This visualization promotes mental relaxation and can be a powerful tool for stress reduction. It's also useful for stimulating creativity and can offer a pleasant mental escape for those with physical movement limitations.

Exercise: Beach Visualization

How to Do It: Sit comfortably and close your eyes. Inhale deeply, envisioning yourself in a peaceful beach setting. Visualize the waves gently breaking on the shore, feel the warm sand under your feet, the sun on your skin, and the breeze in your hair. Spend several minutes in this visualization, letting the peacefulness of the scene fill you.

Benefits: This exercise is excellent for reducing stress and anxiety. It's also beneficial for those who feel confined or restricted, as it provides a mental escape to a serene environment.

Exercise: Forest Walk Visualization

How to Do It: Sit in a comfortable position and close your eyes. Imagine walking through a lush, green forest. Visualize the tall trees, hear the sound of leaves rustling, and feel the soft ground beneath your feet. Notice the scents of the forest and the cool, fresh air. Continue this walk in your mind, feeling the peace and serenity of the forest envelop you.

Benefits: This visualization promotes relaxation and mental tranquility. It can be particularly soothing for those who find calm in nature and for those seeking an escape from urban or indoor environments.

Each exercise deepens the Chair Yoga experience, making it much more than a physical practice. By incorporating these elements, practitioners can enjoy a more comprehensive approach to well-being, engaging body, mind, and spirit in a harmonious and healing journey.

Chapter 4: The Power of Yoga Mudras

Introducing to Yoga Mudras and Their Benefits

Welcome to Chapter 4, a chapter that unfolds like an ancient tome, revealing the enigmatic world of Yoga Mudras. These symbolic gestures, born from the ancient wisdom of yoga, offer a profound and transformative experience, especially for those who are gracefully sailing through the serene waters of their golden years. Let us guide you through this universe of silent gestures, telling stories of energy and awareness, and discover how they can enrich your journey in Chair Yoga.

The Essence of Yoga Mudras

The term 'Mudra,' meaning 'seal' or 'gesture' in Sanskrit, holds a universe of meaning and power. These hand gestures are not mere movements; they are keys unlocking doors to new states of consciousness, channeling the flow of energy, and influencing the body's internal systems. By creating specific formations with the fingers and hands, mudras stimulate different parts of the body and mind, enabling practitioners to access specific moods, mindsets, or energies.

The Multifaceted Benefits of Mudras

Especially suitable for Chair Yoga, mudras add an active element to the practice, ensuring that hands and fingers, which are connected to various parts of the brain and body, remain engaged and stimulated. The benefits of mudras are manifold:

- **Holistic Wellbeing:** Mudras help balance the five elements (earth, water, fire, air, and ether) in the body, leading to physical and mental equilibrium.
- **Enhanced Concentration:** Certain mudras are designed to increase focus and mental acuity.
- **Energy Regulation:** Mudras regulate and redirect the body's energy flow, aiding in rejuvenation and vitality.
- **Emotional Balance:** Mudras can influence emotional states, helping to alleviate feelings of stress, anxiety, or depression.
- **Therapeutic Benefits:** Many mudras offer therapeutic benefits, aiding in ailments ranging from insomnia to cardiac problems.

Incorporating Mudras Into Your Chair Yoga Practice: A Holistic Approach

In the peaceful universe of Chair Yoga, especially for those in their golden years, mudras reveal themselves as precious keys to a deeper and more holistic practice. These hand gestures, transcending mere physical expression, are subtle yet powerful tools that harmonize the body's postures with yoga's mental and spiritual dimensions.

Imagine a yoga posture as a charming melody. Now, add a mudra to this melody, and you'll enrich its harmony. Mudras elevate the physical aspects of Chair Yoga by adding an energetic and spiritual dimension that amplifies the benefits and depth of each movement. While the body finds stability in a seated position, mudras offer a focus point for the mind, deepening the meditative aspects of the practice for a richer, more introspective experience.

Moreover, mudras align the physical practice of Chair Yoga with spiritual intentions, acting as silent yet potent communicators that express and channel our deepest aspirations and inner energies.

In this book, we'll take you on a journey where mudras are skillfully woven into various Chair Yoga practices. These symbolic gestures are naturally integrated into breathing techniques, warm-up exercises, and complete routines, making the Chair Yoga experience even richer and more comprehensive. This integration aims to make Chair Yoga a complete physical experience and transforms the practice into a holistic journey involving mind, body, and spirit.

Through the use of mudras, each session becomes an opportunity to unite physical movement and spiritual intention, reminding us that every gesture, every breath, and every posture carries the potential for profound transformation at all levels: physical, mental, and spiritual. By incorporating mudras into your Chair Yoga practice, you embark on a journey that transcends physical limitations, creating a sanctuary where restoration and progress happen, touching not just the physical self but echoing through every aspect of who you are.

Ultimately, Chair Yoga with mudras is not just a path to maintain physical fitness; it's a way to nurture a balanced, harmonious, and enriched life in every aspect.

Here are some ideas on how you can integrate mudras into your Chair Yoga practice

- **During breathing exercises:** Mudras can be used during breathing exercises to intensify their effects. For instance, the Gyan Mudra can be paired with deep breathing techniques to promote mental calmness and concentration.
- **In the warm-up:** Including mudras in warm-up exercises helps set the intention and awareness for the session. A mudra like the Anjali Mudra can be used at the beginning of the practice to create a moment of inner connection and gratitude.
- **In complete routines:** During Chair Yoga sequences, you can pair specific mudras with certain postures to amplify their benefits.

By incorporating mudras into the various practices described in this book, you'll experience a unique synergy between movement, breath, and intention. It not only makes Chair Yoga a complete physical practice but also transforms it into a rich, multidimensional journey that engages the mind, body, and spirit.

The Bridge Between Movement and Intent

They remind us that every gesture, every breath, and every posture holds the possibility for significant change and growth, affecting us not only physically but also mentally and spiritually.

A Journey of Holistic Wellbeing

Introducing mudras into your Chair Yoga routine invites you on an expansive journey beyond the boundaries of the physical form. You open up a space where healing and growth occur not just on a bodily level, but resonate through every layer of your being. This approach ensures that your journey in Chair Yoga isn't just about maintaining physical fitness; it's about nurturing a balanced, harmonious, and enriched life.

With each mudra woven into your sessions, you can connect more deeply with yourself and the universe. Whether you're seeking a moment of tranquility or invigorating energy, mudras offer a pathway to explore and embrace these states. It's a journey that celebrates both the body and its agility and the mind and spirit in their quest for balance and serenity.

Every movement in Chair Yoga, enriched with the depth of mudras, becomes a dance between the visible and the invisible, a dialogue between the physical and the ethereal. It's a practice that transcends mere exercise, becoming an art that elevates the entirety of your being, a journey where every step is a step towards a more fulfilling and satisfying life.

In the Journey of Mudras: Ten Timeless Gestures in Chair Yoga

Chair Yoga isn't just a series of seated postures; it's a journey into the depths of self-awareness and energy management. Mudras, with their subtle yet profound power, play a pivotal role in this exploration. They aren't just simple hand gestures; they are keys that unlock various aspects of our physical, mental, and spiritual well-being. Let's dive into ten timeless mudras together and understand how they can enrich your Chair Yoga practice.

Anjali Mudra (Seal of Salutation)

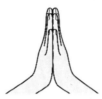

Description: The Anjali Mudra involves bringing your palms together at the heart center, fingers extended upward. This gesture is often associated with greeting, prayer, and respect in various cultures, especially in Indian traditions.

Benefits: The Anjali Mudra promotes a sense of balance, focus, and inner harmony. It symbolizes gratitude, respect, and a connection with oneself and others. In Chair Yoga, especially for those in their golden years, this mudra helps center the mind, encouraging a state of calmness and introspection. It's a gesture that nurtures a feeling of devotion and reverence, both in a spiritual context and in self-respect.

Incorporating the Anjali Mudra into Chair Yoga sessions can be a powerful tool for grounding and centering at the beginning or end of a practice. It brings a moment of pause and reflection, allowing practitioners to connect with their inner selves and the present moment deeply. This mudra also serves as a reminder of the interconnectedness of all beings and can be a symbol of offering gratitude for the body, the practice, and the wisdom that comes with age.

Using the Anjali Mudra during meditation or breathing exercises can enhance the sense of serenity and focus. It's a simple yet profound gesture that embodies humility, respect, and a balanced state of mind, making it an essential element in the practice of Chair Yoga for those embracing their golden years.

Kali Mudra (Seal of Transformation)

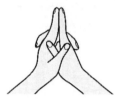

Description: To perform the Kali Mudra, interlace your fingers while extending just your index fingers, which touch each other. The intertwined fingers symbolize the merging of different energies, and the extended index fingers represent clarity and direction.

Benefits: Named after the Hindu goddess Kali, known for her power to conquer darkness and bring about transformation, the Kali Mudra channels energies of change and self-affirmation. It's particularly beneficial during times of change or when seeking to overcome obstacles and fears.

Incorporating the Kali Mudra into Chair Yoga sessions can help focus intentions and energies towards change, strength, and overcoming external and internal barriers. Within the context of Chair Yoga, this mudra can empower seniors, especially when facing the challenges that come with aging. It can also be used to channel inner strength and determination during practice, promoting a mindset of overcoming limitations and embracing change with confidence.

Tattva Mudra (Seal of Truth)

Description: The Tattva Mudra, or Seal of Truth, embodies honesty, authenticity, and a commitment to living one's truth. The specific formation of this mudra may vary, but it often involves a distinct positioning of the fingers, symbolizing speaking and living truthfully.

Benefits: The Tattva Mudra is known for its ability to help individuals align with their true selves and express their deepest thoughts and feelings with honesty and integrity. It encourages practitioners to embrace authenticity in their actions and words, fostering a sense of inner peace and alignment with personal values and principles.

In the context of Chair Yoga for seniors, the Tattva Mudra can be a powerful tool for self-reflection and introspection. It aids in exploring personal beliefs, values, and experiences, helping cultivate self-awareness and personal integrity. This mudra is particularly beneficial in meditative practices focused on self-discovery and personal growth.

Incorporating the Tattva Mudra into Chair Yoga sessions can involve using it during quiet contemplation or meditation moments. It serves as a gentle reminder to stay truthful and authentic in one's journey, both on and off the yoga mat. For seniors, this practice offers a way to connect with their wisdom and experiences, honoring their life's journey with honesty and grace. The Tattva Mudra thus becomes not just a physical gesture, but a symbol of living a life of truth and authenticity, essential elements for holistic well-being.

Vayu Mudra (Seal of Air)

Description: The Vayu Mudra, or Seal of Air, is achieved by folding the index finger towards the base of the thumb and then pressing it with the thumb while the other fingers stay straight and relaxed. This gesture relates to the air element in the body.

Benefits: The Vayu Mudra is especially beneficial for regulating and balancing air-related conditions within the body. It's known to help alleviate symptoms of excess air, such as flatulence, bloating, and joint discomfort. By reducing the air element in the body, this mudra can also bring a sense of calm and stability to the mind.

In Chair Yoga practices, especially for seniors, the Vayu Mudra can be a gentle yet effective way to address digestive issues and joint pain, which are common in older age. The mudra can be incorporated into sessions focusing on gentle movements and breathing exercises, enhancing the overall benefits of the practice.

Using the Vayu Mudra during Chair Yoga sessions simply involves adopting the gesture while seated comfortably, whether during meditation, breathwork, or even gentle stretches and movements. Its ease of execution makes it an accessible tool for seniors, providing them with a simple way to manage and alleviate discomfort related to air imbalances. The Vayu Mudra thus becomes a valuable addition to the Chair Yoga routine, offering both physical relief and mental tranquility.

Vitarka Mudra (Seal of Teaching or Discussion)

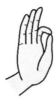

Description: The Vitarka Mudra is a gesture of teaching and discussion. To perform it, form a circle with your thumb and index finger, keeping the other fingers extended upwards. This circle symbolizes the continuous flow of energy and the transmission of wisdom. The gesture can be made with one or both hands and is often depicted in images of Buddha and other deities imparting wisdom.

Benefits: The Vitarka Mudra is associated with intellectual discussion, teaching, and debate. It promotes a clear and open mind, facilitates communication, and encourages knowledge sharing. This mudra can be particularly beneficial for seniors engaged in learning, teaching, or intellectual pursuits, as it helps to stimulate the mind and aids in expressing ideas and thoughts.

Incorporating the Vitarka Mudra into Chair Yoga practices, especially for those in their golden years, can be a powerful way to encourage mental clarity and the exchange of wisdom. It can be used during moments of discussion or reflection within a yoga class or even during personal study or contemplation.

The Vitarka Mudra serves as a reminder of the importance of continuous learning and sharing knowledge. For seniors, this mudra can symbolize a lifetime of experience and wisdom, and the ongoing journey of learning and teaching. When combined with focused breathing and meditation, the Vitarka Mudra can deepen the sense of connection to one's intellectual and communicative abilities, enhancing both personal growth and the sharing of knowledge within a community. This mudra is not just a physical gesture but a symbol of the endless cycle of learning, teaching, and growth that continues throughout life.

Lotus Mudra (Seal of Purity and Enlightenment)

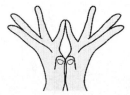

Description: The Lotus Mudra, a symbol of purity and enlightenment, mirrors the blooming of a lotus flower. To perform this mudra, bring your hands together in front of your chest, touching at the base of the palms and the tips of your little and thumb fingers while the other fingers spread apart like the petals of a blooming lotus. This mudra is often held at the heart center, signifying the opening of the heart and the awakening of the purest form of consciousness.

Benefits: The Lotus Mudra is especially beneficial in evoking feelings of purity and peace within the practitioner. It aids in opening the heart chakra, promoting sentiments of love, compassion, and connection. This mudra is often used to encourage an awareness of inner sanctity and to remind practitioners of their inherent beauty and grace, much like a lotus flower blossoming in muddy waters yet remaining unstained.

Incorporating the Lotus Mudra into Chair Yoga routines, especially for those in their golden years, can be a powerful way to enhance the spiritual and emotional aspects of the practice. It can be utilized during quiet contemplation or meditation moments, helping foster a deeper connection with oneself and the surrounding world. The Lotus Mudra is a reminder of the resilience and purity of the human spirit, encouraging practitioners to rise above challenges and embrace their journey with openness and grace. With its serene symbolism, this mudra brings profound depth to the Chair Yoga experience, nurturing the soul and uplifting the mind.

Mushti Mudra (Seal of Release and Letting Go)

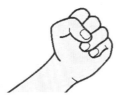

Description: The Mushti Mudra is a gesture of release and liberation. To execute this mudra, clench both hands into fists, placing the thumbs over the fingers, not tucked inside. This gesture of grasping and then releasing symbolizes capturing negative energies or emotions and then letting go or shedding these burdens.

Benefits: The Mushti Mudra is especially useful for releasing repressed emotions, stress, or anger. It aids in the process of emotional cleansing, helping to release unnecessary or harmful tensions accumulated in the body and mind. This mudra is also known to assist digestion and improve energy flow (prana) within the body.

Incorporating the Mushti Mudra into Chair Yoga practices, particularly for those in their golden years, can provide a powerful tool for emotional equilibrium. It can be used in sequences where the intention is to let go of the past, disperse negative energies, or simply find a sense of emotional release. This mudra can be particularly effective when combined with deep breathing exercises, where each exhale symbolizes the shedding of tension and negative emotions.

The Mushti Mudra is more than just a physical gesture; it's a symbolic act of opening to new possibilities and freeing oneself from the chains of negative emotions. For senior practitioners, this mudra can be especially meaningful, offering a way to let go of longstanding burdens and embrace the present moment with a lighter heart and a clearer mind. Practicing this mudra in Chair Yoga sessions can be a liberating experience, bringing a sense of renewal and emotional freedom.

Dhyana Mudra (Seal of Meditation)

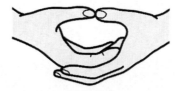

Description: The Dhyana Mudra, or Seal of Meditation, is a classic gesture for meditation and contemplation. To perform this mudra, place both hands in your lap, one on top of the other with palms facing upward. The thumbs of both hands gently touch at the tips, creating a subtle and elegant oval shape. This mudra is often associated with deep meditative states and spiritual awakening.

Benefits: The Dhyana Mudra is renowned for enhancing meditation and contemplation. It fosters a sense of inner peace, calmness, and mental clarity. By adopting this mudra during meditation or relaxation practices in Chair Yoga, practitioners can deepen their experience, finding a more profound connection with their inner self. It is particularly beneficial for seniors as it aids in reducing stress, calming the mind, and fostering a state of serene mindfulness.

Incorporating the Dhyana Mudra into Chair Yoga routines, especially for those in their later years, provides a simple yet powerful tool to enhance the meditative aspects of the practice. This mudra can be used at the beginning or end of a yoga session to help center the mind and prepare for deeper relaxation. It's also effective when used in standalone meditation practices, enabling the practitioner to delve into deeper states of tranquility and self-awareness. With its graceful form and profound impact, the Dhyana Mudra adds a layer of spiritual richness to the Chair Yoga experience, encouraging a balanced and harmonious state of being.

Apana Mudra (Seal of Digestion)

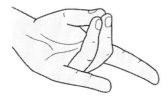

Description: The Apana Mudra is created by connecting the thumb to the tips of the middle and ring fingers while keeping the other fingers extended. This gesture, usually performed with both hands, is known for its grounding and calming properties.

Benefits: The Apana Mudra is particularly beneficial for promoting healthy digestion and aiding in the body's detoxification processes. It's believed to stimulate the Apana Vayu, one of the five pranas or vital forces in the body, responsible for waste elimination and regulating the digestive system. Regular practice of this mudra can help alleviate digestive issues, improve bowel movements, and assist in the overall cleansing of the body.

For seniors practicing Chair Yoga, the Apana Mudra can be a gentle yet effective way to support digestive health, which is often a concern in later years. It also helps create a sense of balance and grounding, making it suitable for practices aimed at stabilizing energy and calming the mind.

Incorporating the Apana Mudra into Chair Yoga routines can be done during breathing exercises, particularly those focused on abdominal breathing, or during meditation sessions to enhance focus on the lower abdomen and promote a sense of internal cleansing. This mudra serves as a subtle reminder of the importance of nurturing the body's natural elimination processes and maintaining a healthy digestive system, contributing to overall well-being and vitality in the golden years.

Jala Mudra (Seal of Water)

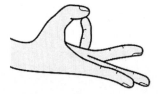

Description: To perform the Jala Mudra, touch the tip of your little finger to the tip of your thumb, with the other three fingers extended straight. This mudra resembles a gesture that is gentle yet flowing, much like the qualities of water.

Benefits: Jala, in Sanskrit, means 'water', and this mudra is dedicated to balancing the water element within the body. It is particularly beneficial for hydrating cells and tissues and is often used to combat issues related to dryness, such as dry skin or dehydration. For seniors practicing Chair Yoga, the Jala Mudra can be a soothing and nurturing gesture, reminding them of the fluidity and adaptability of water. This mudra helps maintain moisture balance in the body, which can be essential for overall health and well-being, especially in older age. Additionally, it encourages a sense of calmness and emotional fluidity, helping to ease feelings of rigidity or stiffness, both physically and mentally. Integrating the Jala Mudra into Chair Yoga routines can aid in cultivating a sense of ease and smooth flow in movements and breath, mirroring water's serene and life-sustaining qualities.

Incorporating these mudras into your Chair Yoga routine adds an enriching layer to the practice. They offer a unique way to engage the subtle energies of the body and mind, leading to a more rounded and fulfilling yoga experience. Whether you want to enhance physical health, mental clarity, or spiritual depth, these mudras can be valuable tools in your Chair Yoga journey. Remember, the beauty of Chair Yoga lies not only in its accessibility but also in its capacity to be a holistic practice, addressing your entire being.

Chapter 5: Gentle Warm-Up and Cooldown

In the enchanting realm of Chair Yoga, the significance of a thoughtful warmup and the importance of a mindful cooldown hold paramount importance, much like the overture and finale of a delightful symphony. This chapter delves deep into the essentials of these practices, ensuring a yoga experience that's as safe and effective as it is enjoyable.

The Art of Warming Up

Imagine beginning a Chair Yoga session without a proper warmup—it's like starting a car on a frosty morning without giving the engine a chance to warm up. Here's why a gentle warmup is so crucial:

- **Enhancing flexibility and mobility:** Warmup exercises in Chair Yoga are like a gentle invitation to your muscles and joints, preparing them for the journey ahead. They gradually increase blood flow, making your muscles more supple and less prone to injury.
- **Mental tuning:** It's like tuning an instrument before a concert. Warmup exercises help tune your mind for the session, offering a transition from the hustle and bustle of daily life to a more reflective, meditative state.
- **Breathing and heart rate regulation:** These exercises gradually elevate your heart rate and introduce deeper, more rhythmic breathing, essential for efficient oxygen delivery during your yoga practice.
- **Awareness of physical limits:** Warmups are like a gentle conversation with your body, helping you understand its capabilities and limits on any given day. This awareness is key in tailoring your yoga practice to suit your current physical state.

Warm Up Practices

Breath Awareness With Anjali Mudra

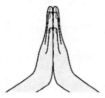

Setting the Scene: Begin by sitting comfortably in your chair, feeling the support beneath you. Place your palms together in front of your chest in Anjali Mudra, with your fingers extended upwards, forming a prayer-like position.

The Practice: Close your eyes, tuning into your natural breathing pattern, alongside the balance and focus the Anjali Mudra cultivates. Let your breaths deepen gradually, feeling the gentle wave of calmness washing over you.

The Duration: Spend a few minutes in this state, harmonizing your mind and body, preparing for the journey ahead with a sense of gratitude and centeredness.

Neck Stretches With Vayu Mudra

Getting Comfortable: Sit upright, shoulders relaxed. Form the Vayu Mudra by folding the index fingers towards the thumbs' bases and pressing them down, other fingers extended.

The Movement: Tilt your head gently to each side, feeling the stretch along your neck, the Vayu Mudra enhancing balance and relief in the area.

The Finish: Rotate your neck in smooth, circular motions, maintaining the mudra to release tension and bring calmness to your mind.

Shoulder Rolls With Mushti Mudra

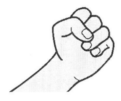

The Setup: Begin with a playful shrug of your shoulders, lifting them towards your ears.

The Action: As you roll your shoulders, form the Mushti Mudra by making gentle fists, symbolizing the release of stored emotions. Reverse the direction, feeling the emotional release with each rotation.

Arm and Wrist Circles With Lotus Mudra

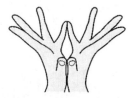

The Extension: Stretch your arms outward, invoking the grace of wings ready to take flight.

The Movement: As you rotate your wrists, transition into the Lotus Mudra, fingertips of thumbs and little fingers touching, other fingers spread like a blooming lotus, enhancing the fluidity and openness of the movements.

Gentle Spinal Twists With Dhyana Mudra

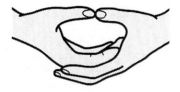

The Alignment: Sit tall, one hand on the opposite knee, the other behind you for support.

The Twist: As you rotate your torso, adopt the Dhyana Mudra in your lap, one hand atop the other, palms up, thumbs touching, forming an elegant oval. The twist, combined with the mudra, deepens your sense of inner peace and contemplation.

These warmup practices aren't just exercises; they're an intimate dialogue with your body, a way to tune in and set the tone for your Chair Yoga session. With each movement and breath, you pave the way for a more mindful and rewarding practice.

The Grace of Cooling Down

Cooling down after Chair Yoga is like savoring a sweet dessert after a satisfying meal. Here's why it's an essential phase of your practice:

- **Preventing dizziness and discomfort:** Just like easing off a merry-go-round, cooling down helps in gradually bringing your heart rate and blood pressure back to resting levels, preventing dizziness or discomfort.
- **Muscle recovery and flexibility:** It's a time for your muscles to unwind and relax, reducing postexercise soreness and enhancing overall flexibility over time.
- **Reflection and absorption:** This phase is your moment to reflect on the practice, bask in its benefits, and extend that sense of calm and accomplishment beyond the session.
- **Transition back to daily life:** Just as a good book gently brings you back to reality from its pages, cooling down eases you back into the rhythm of daily life, allowing you to carry the tranquility and mindfulness from the session into your everyday activities.

In summary, Chapter 5 highlights the importance of gentle warmups and cooldowns in Chair Yoga. These practices are not mere physical routines; they are integral to a holistic yoga experience, bridging your yoga practice with everyday life, and ensuring a journey that is as nurturing as it is enriching.

Cooldown Practices

In the serene world of Chair Yoga, cooling down practices are like the gentle lullaby after an invigorating day, essential to complete your yoga journey. Let's explore the art of unwinding with these calming exercises:

Deep Breathing With Apana Mudra

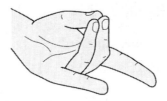

Setting the tone: As you return to breath awareness, form the Apana Mudra by connecting your thumbs to the tips of the middle and ring fingers, other fingers extended, enhancing your focus on decelerating your breath.

The practice: Inhale deeply through your nose, feeling the grounding energy of the Apana Mudra. Exhale slowly through your mouth, feeling a sense of release and detoxification with every breath out.

Forward Bend With Jala Mudra

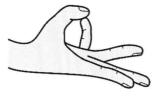

Beginning the descent: Seated in your chair, take a deep breath in, and gently lift your arms skyward, embracing the space above. Integrate the Jala Mudra by touching the tips of your little fingers to the thumbs, other fingers extended, as you breathe in and lift your arms.

The dive: As you exhale and fold forward, maintain the Jala Mudra, symbolizing the fluidity and adaptability of water, as your hands drift towards your feet.

Seated Cat-Cow Stretches With Kali Mudra

Finding fluidity: As you place your hands on your knees, transition into the Kali Mudra by interlacing your fingers except for the extended index fingers.

The dance: Move through the Cat-Cow sequence, rounding your back and drawing your chin inward, with the Kali Mudra, embodying strength and transformation, empowering your spine's flexibility.

Seated Ankle Rolls and Point-Flex With Mushti Mudra

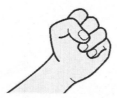

The flow: Extend one leg out, leading with the heel, then the toes, as if painting circles in the air with your foot. Form the Mushti Mudra by gently making a fist, releasing any pent-up emotions with each rotation and flex.

The release: Rotate your ankle in gentle swirls, then alternate between pointing and flexing your foot, like the rise and fall of ocean waves. Maintain the Mushti Mudra, feeling emotional release and rejuvenation in your lower extremities.

Meditation or Guided Relaxation with Dhyana Mudra

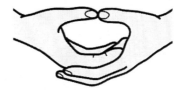

The quietude: Settle into a state of meditation or guided relaxation, adopting the Dhyana Mudra, hands in your lap, one on top of the other, thumbs touching, facilitating deeper meditative states.

The journey inward: As you relax each body part, let the Dhyana Mudra guide you into profound tranquility and self-awareness.

The gratitude: In this state of deep relaxation, let the mudra remind you of the peace and wisdom cultivated through your practice.

Remember, the key is to move gently and mindfully, honoring your body's boundaries and using these moments to deeply connect with your inner self. These practices not only prepare and restore your body but also contribute to an overall sense of well-being and balance.

Chapter 6: Seated Poses for Strength, Flexibility, and Balance

A Variety of Seated Yoga Poses

Welcome to a transformative journey through the art of yoga routines. In this chapter, we delve into the significance and myriad benefits that structured yoga routines offer to practitioners at all levels, with special attention to beginners and those in their golden years. Whether you're new to the world of yoga or searching for a practice that prioritizes stability and safety over complex poses, this chapter has something precious to offer you.

Here, you will find carefully selected routines specifically designed for beginners and those who favor seated positions. These routines introduce you to essential poses, breathing techniques, and alignment principles that are both gentle and effective.

Our chapter is designed to meet the needs of those who may not feel confident with standing poses or who wish to prioritize stability and safety in their practice. These seated poses provide numerous benefits, including improved flexibility, enhanced posture, and stress relief, making them perfect for beginners and those in their golden years.

The Benefits of Structured Yoga Routines

- **Consistency:** Routines offer a structured approach, fostering regularity in your practice.
- **Progression:** With routines tailored for beginners and older adults, you can progressively challenge yourself while prioritizing safety and stability.
- **Holistic development:** Yoga routines holistically address physical, mental, and emotional well-being. They enhance flexibility, strength, balance, and inner peace.

- **Time efficiency:** Routines are time-efficient, making it easier to incorporate yoga into your daily life, even amidst a busy schedule.
- **Goal-oriented:** Whether your goal is relaxation, fitness, or improved well-being, these routines can be customized to align with your objectives.

Each routine is designed to be 15 minutes long, featuring six poses. However, it is important to listen to your body. If you find it challenging to maintain a pose for the indicated time, do not worry. Hold each pose for as long as you feel comfortable, and with practice, you will gradually increase your endurance. There is no rush and no pressure—your comfort and safety are the most important.

Routine 1

Mountain Pose Chair

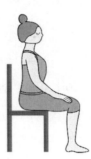

The Mountain Pose offers a host of benefits, including better posture, stronger core muscles, and heightened breath awareness. It acts as an anchor of stability and mindfulness, making it particularly advantageous for beginners and anyone looking to solidify their basic yoga practice. And the best part? There are no specific contraindications associated with this pose, especially when comfortably performed on a chair.

Steps (2 minutes)

1. Start your session by settling into a chair, ensuring your feet are securely positioned on the floor. Place your hands on your thighs, maintain a straight posture, and softly close your eyes.
2. In this seated position, akin to the Mountain Pose Chair, start with your breathing practice. Inhale and exhale deeply a couple of times to establish a serene rhythm.
3. Next, place your palms on your body in the Apana Mudra (see p. 41), right hand over your belly and left hand over your chest. This gesture enhances your focus on the breath, deepening your connection to the body's movements.
  Stay mindful of the rise and fall of your abdomen and chest as you breathe. Continue this focused breathing for 2 minutes, allowing yourself to become more attuned to your body's natural rhythm.

All pose images are copyright by Tummee - sequencing platform for yoga teachers

Hands Chest Chair

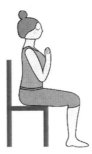

In the Hands Chest Chair Yoga Pose, the practitioner sits comfortably on a chair, with a straight back and feet firmly grounded. The hands are brought to chest level, palms facing each other, either held close together or with a slight gap between them.

The elbows are bent and point outward, roughly parallel to the ground. This pose helps to open the chest, offering a gentle stretch to the chest muscles and the front part of the shoulders.

The Hands Chest Chair pose, with hands at the heart in Anjali Mudra, serves as a universal gateway to calmness and focus. It's easily adaptable and a haven in daily routines, offering a momentary escape to connect with one's breath. As a transitional pose in Chair Yoga, it's a therapeutic tool for those in need of healing, especially post-surgery or trauma. It sets the stage for meditation and pranayama sessions, grounding participants in the present. In our world full of distractions, it strengthens focus and rejuvenates the mind, turning work from mere tasks into joyful endeavors. It is more than a posture; it is a symbol of conscious living.

The simplicity of the Hands Chest Chair Pose makes it widely accessible, but a few considerations ensure its safe practice. Individuals with recent wrist or arm injuries should be cautious about the duration they hold this pose to avoid aggravating their condition. Similarly, those recovering from chronic back issues or recent surgeries should be mindful of the time spent in this seated position to avoid strain. If prolonged sitting causes discomfort in the back, neck, or shoulders, using a rolled blanket for back support can offer relief, ensuring the pose remains comfortable.

Steps (3 minutes)

1. Start by positioning yourself on a chair, making sure your back is erect and your feet are firmly planted on the ground.
2. Take a deep breath in, bring your palms together in Anjali Mudra (see p. 33), and place them against your chest.
3. Allow your elbows to extend outward from your torso in a relaxed manner, ensuring there's no tension in your fingers, wrists, or shoulders.
4. If comfortable, gently close your eyes and focus on deep, even breaths. Feel the rhythm of your body as it responds to each inhalation and exhalation.
5. Let any fleeting thoughts come and go without resistance. As you center your attention on your breath, these thoughts will naturally dissipate. Stay in the Hands Chest Chair pose for at least 3 minutes or as long as you feel comfortable.
6. To conclude the pose, gradually open your eyes, release your arms, and move on to the next practice.

Three-Part Breath Chair

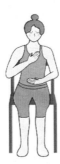

Welcome to the meditative and warming practice of the Three-Part Breath Chair Pose, a delightful journey mostly experienced while comfortably seated. Imagine this pose as a conductor of breath, guiding the energy flow through every corner of your body. Here, you, the practitioner, will focus on a breathing technique that engages three distinct body parts, heightening your awareness and prepping you for more dynamic poses. This pose is especially handy for grounding and centering your mind. Its gentle nature makes it a staple in Chair Yoga sequences and even in prenatal yoga.

The Three-Part Breath Chair Pose is akin to a rich reservoir of benefits. Focusing on deep, three-part breathing amps up your oxygen intake, which is like giving your lungs a health boost. This focus on breath does wonders for your mind too, slicing through stress and sharpening mental clarity while energizing every bit of you. As a warm-up pose, it lays down a solid foundation, getting you physically and mentally ready for the yoga adventure ahead. Plus, it's a great way to tune into your breathing patterns, fostering a deep bond between your body and mind.

Now, a little word of caution with the Three-Part Breath Chair Pose. If you've recently had surgery, especially around your chest or belly, do have a chat with your doctor before diving in. For those with breathing challenges like asthma, it's best to practice under expert eyes to keep things comfy for your lungs. And, though the pose is generally gentle, if you've got a fussy back, proceed with care and maybe grab a supportive prop.

Steps (3 minutes)

1. Start by sitting snugly on a chair, back straight as an arrow, feet firmly on the ground.
2. Place one hand on your heart and the other on your belly, adopting the Vayu Mudra (see p. 36) with each hand. As you position your hands, feel the connection between your breath and the gentle gesture of the mudra, enhancing your focus and relaxation.
3. Breathe deeply through your nose, letting only your diaphragm lift—keep that chest still. Feel your belly hand rise.
4. Keep that inhale going into your rib cage, feel it expand, and your chest lift–up goes the chest hand too.
5. Finish that inhale into the upper chest, right below your collarbone.
6. Exhale nice and slow through your nose, feeling each section—upper chest, ribcage, and belly—gently fall.
7. Keep this three-part breathing going for 3 minutes, focusing on each segment.
8. After 3 minutes, let your breath flow naturally and just notice any shifts in how you feel, physically or emotionally.

Pigeon Pose Chair

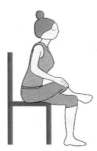

The Pigeon Pose Chair is a thorough exercise encompassing various muscle groups. It intricately involves the feet, ankles, glutes, hamstrings, and hips, with a special emphasis on external hip rotation. This versatility makes it a key component in a range of yoga sequences, including chair yoga, prenatal yoga, and hip-opening sequences.

The benefits of the Pigeon Pose Chair are diverse. It stretches and strengthens essential areas, alleviating rigidity and fostering a more flexible and comfortable lower body. The pose also has a unique emotional dimension, potentially aiding in the release of negative energy and fostering emotional balance, especially beneficial for hips often burdened with stress and tension.

Additionally, the pose possesses therapeutic qualities, particularly effective in relieving discomforts like sciatic nerve pain by stretching the hip flexors and glutes. For our seasoned yoga enthusiasts, this pose not only helps maintain hip mobility but also enhances their meditation practices by increasing comfort in seated positions.

As a preparatory pose, the Pigeon Pose Chair conditions the body for more demanding positions, ensuring minimal strain on sensitive areas such as the knees and ankles. It's also a valuable practice for those managing osteoporosis, athletes in recovery, and even office workers or travelers looking for a quick, beneficial stretch.

However, it's crucial to recognize the contraindications. Those with injuries or recent surgeries in the ankle, foot, or hip areas, or individuals with conditions like fibromyalgia or coccydynia, should avoid this pose. Our seasoned practitioners should approach this practice with caution and under proper guidance to ensure safety and maximize benefits.

Steps (2 minutes)

1. Start by sitting comfortably.
2. Inhale, and gently lift your right leg with your hands.
3. Place your right leg over your left thigh, ensuring you remain seated comfortably.
4. Focus on flexing your hip joint and knee to maintain fitness and flexibility.
5. Once your leg is comfortably positioned, try sitting up straight and take two deep breaths. Hold this position for 2 minutes.
6. If it's challenging to place one leg over the other, simply lift your right leg, hold it in your arms for a few moments, and then gradually release it.
7. While performing these steps, position your hands in the Tattva Mudra (see p. 35).

Cow Pose Chair

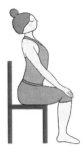

The Cow Pose Chair variation is a seated adaptation of the traditional Cow Pose, crafted to bring flexibility and movement to the spine while you're comfortably seated. Imagine yourself sitting upright in a chair, feet firmly planted on the ground. As you inhale, you gently arch your back, nudging your chest forward and lifting your chin just a tad, creating a gentle concave shape in your upper body. This movement gives a nice stretch and activates the lower and upper back, chest, pelvic area, and those often-forgotten psoas muscles. Think of it as a warm-up act, preparing your body for more challenging postures or sequences. You'll find this pose a regular in Chair Yoga and prenatal yoga sequences, particularly those focusing on heart openings.

The Cow Pose Chair is a treasure trove of benefits, primarily focusing on spinal health. Its arching motion is like a loving hug for your spine, boosting its flexibility and breathing new life into your lower and upper back. As you push your chest forward in this pose, there's a real sense of opening up across the chest muscles – a godsend for those of us who spend hours hunched over desks. The seated nature of this pose, combined with a deliberate tilt of the pelvis during the arch, gives a lovely stretch and strengthens the pelvic muscles, key players in our core strength. And let's not forget the gentle stretch to the psoas muscles, crucial for our core stability and overall posture.

All pose images are copyright by Tummee - sequencing platform for yoga teachers

On the flip side, while the Cow Pose Chair is renowned for its safety and adaptability, a word of caution is in order. Those who've recently had back injuries or have underlying spine issues should approach with care. It might be wiser to skip this pose or to do it under the guidance of a seasoned yoga instructor. And for those with a sensitive neck, remember not to strain it when lifting the chin during the pose. In all yoga practices, the golden rule remains: always listen to your body's signals and steer clear of movements that cause pain or significant discomfort.

Steps (3 minutes)

1. Comfortably sit on a chair, feet flat on the ground.
2. Place your hands on your knees or thighs. In each hand, form the Vitarka Mudra (see p. 37).
3. Take a deep breath, arching your back and pushing your chest and stomach forward. Maintain the Vitarka Mudra on your thighs.
4. Slightly lift your chin, allowing your head to tilt back gently, but be mindful not to strain your neck.
5. Exhale and return to the starting position with a neutral spine, keeping your hands with Vitarka Mudra on your thighs.
6. Repeat this movement for 3 minutes, syncing it with your breath. As you move through the arching of your back, keep your hands steady in the Vitarka Mudra, allowing the gesture to aid in maintaining focus and calmness during the pose.

Mountain Pose Heel Raised Chair

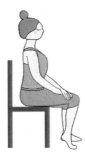

In the Mountain Pose with Heels Raised, you sit upright in a chair, keeping your back straight and your feet firmly on the ground. As the name suggests, in this variation, you lift your heels off the floor, engaging those calf muscles and bringing more awareness to your lower legs. Your hands can either rest comfortably on your thighs or be raised above your head, lining up with your ears. Remember to keep your breathing steady and even all the way through.

The Mountain Pose with Heels Raised comes with many benefits. Lifting your heels not only engages and strengthens the calf muscles but can also wake up the arches of your feet. This variation offers a gentle stretch to your Achilles tendon and might just improve your balance and body awareness in space. Plus, the upright posture helps keep your spine straight, aiding in better overall posture and maybe even easing some of that pesky back discomfort. Lifting your arms also helps stretch out the sides of your body and improve upper body flexibility.

Although it's generally a safe pose, those with recent ankle injuries or balance issues should take a cautious approach to the Mountain Pose with Heels Raised. It's important to make sure your chair is stable to avoid any mishaps. Also, if you have severe back problems, it's wise to check with a healthcare professional before giving this pose a try. It's always crucial to be aware of your own limits and make adjustments as needed.

Steps (2 minutes)

1. Sit upright on a chair, ensuring both feet are flat on the ground and hip-width apart.
2. Keep your spine straight, and your shoulders relaxed.
3. For the hand position, form the Dhyana Mudra (see p. 40).
4. Take a deep breath in and, as you exhale, gently lift your heels off the ground, pressing onto the balls of your feet.
5. Engage your calf muscles and maintain steady breathing. Keep your focus serene, reflecting the tranquility of the Dhyana Mudra.
6. Hold the position for 2 minutes, keeping the heels raised and the spine straight.
7. On an exhale, slowly lower your heels back to the ground.

Relax and take a few breaths in the Dhyana Mudra before repeating the pose or moving on to another one. This mudra should help to deepen your sense of relaxation and focus throughout the exercise.

The Beauty of Yoga Is That

You Can Start Where You Are, As You Are

Routine 1

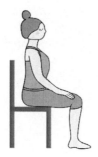 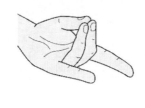

Mountain Pose Chair with Apana Mudra
(2 minutes)

Begin seated in Mountain Pose Chair on a chair with feet flat. Close your eyes and breathe deeply for two breaths. Place the right hand on the belly and the left on the chest, and focus on the breath for 2 minutes.

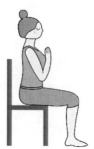 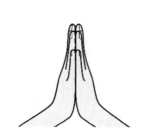

Hands Chest Chair with Anjali Mudra
(3 minutes)

Sit upright on a chair with grounded feet. Join your hands at the chest in the Anjali Mudra position. Extend elbows gently outward, relaxing fingers and shoulders. Close your eyes if comfortable, focusing on deep breaths. Allow thoughts to flow naturally. Hold for 3 minutes or as desired. Slowly open your eyes, release your arms, and transition.

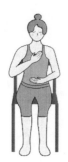 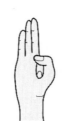

Three-Part Breath Chair with Vayu Mudra
(3 minutes)

Sit on a chair, ensuring your back is erect and your feet grounded. With one hand on your chest and the other on your abdomen, inhale deeply through the nose, feeling the abdomen rise first, then the ribcage, and finally the upper chest. Exhale slowly, observing the gradual fall of each section. Repeat this segmented breathing for 3 minutes, and then return to natural breathing, noting any shifts in your well-being.

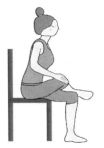 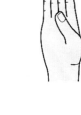

Pigeon Pose Chair with Tattva Mudra
(2 minutes)

Gently, with an inhale, the right leg is lifted by the hands, gracefully crossing it over the left thigh. Ensuring comfort remains paramount in this position. As the leg finds its resting place, the practitioner is encouraged to straighten the spine, embracing the calm for 2 minutes. For those finding the leg cross challenging, a modified approach involves simply cradling the right leg before a slow release.

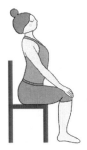 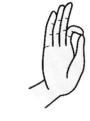

Cow Pose Chair with Vitarka Mudra
(3 minutes)

Sit on a chair with feet flat and hands on thighs. Inhale, arch your back, push your chest forward, and gently tilt your head back. Exhale and return to a neutral position. Repeat, moving with your breath, for 3 minutes.

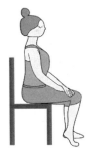 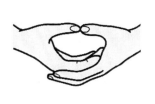

Mountain Pose Heel Raised Chair with Dhyana Mudra
(2 minutes)

Sit upright on a chair with feet flat. As you breathe, lift your heels, pressing onto the balls of your feet. Engage calves and keep the spine straight. Hold this position for 2 minutes, then lower your heels and relax.

Routine 2

Sited Pigeon Pose Palms Up Chair

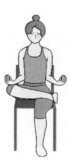

The Seated Pigeon Pose with Palms Up Chair is a gentle adaptation of the traditional Pigeon Pose but is carried out comfortably while sitting in a chair. This variation offers a cozy alternative for those who find the floor pose challenging, making it accessible to practitioners of all levels. With palms facing upwards, this pose helps keep the chest open and fosters a receptive state of mind.

The main focus of the Seated Pigeon Pose with Palms Up Chair is on the hips and the surrounding muscles. By creating external rotation in the hip joint, it provides a deep stretch to the external hip muscles, quadriceps, and even the knees. This pose is especially beneficial for those seeking relief from tight hip muscles, often due to prolonged sitting or standing. Additionally, it helps increase flexibility and mobility in the hip area, making it a favorite in hip-opening sequences.

In terms of benefits, the Seated Pigeon Pose with Palms Up Chair acts as a therapeutic tool for those experiencing tension or stiffness in the hip area. By creating space and promoting blood flow to the region, it can alleviate discomfort and improve overall hip functionality. The pose is also instrumental in enhancing mindfulness, as the palms-up position symbolizes receptivity and openness, inviting practitioners to stay present and connected to their breath and body sensations.

All pose images are copyright by Tummee - sequencing platform for yoga teachers

However, as with all yoga poses, there are certain considerations to keep in mind. Those with acute injuries to the hip, knee, or quadriceps should approach the Seated Pigeon Pose Palms Up Chair cautiously or under the guidance of a qualified yoga instructor. It's essential to ensure proper alignment and to avoid any forceful or abrupt movements, as this can exacerbate any existing conditions. Always prioritize comfort and safety, adjusting the position or using props as needed, and listening to one's body throughout the practice.

Steps (2 minutes)

1. Sit comfortably on a chair with your feet firmly planted on the ground and hip-width apart.
2. Ensure your back is straight.
3. Place your hands on your thighs in the Jala Mudra (see p. 42), and touch the tip of your thumb to the tip of your little finger while the other fingers remain straight.
4. Elevate your right ankle and position it atop your left thigh, forming a figure-four configuration with your limbs.
5. Apply gentle downward pressure on your right knee to enhance the stretch in your hip, taking care to avoid any discomfort.
6. As you hold this pose, focus on the sensation in your hips and the openness of your chest, while maintaining the Jala Mudra with your hands.
7. Maintain the position for 1 minute.
8. Release your right foot back to the ground.
9. Repeat on the opposite side, with the left ankle on the right thigh, continuing to hold the Jala Mudra.

Seated Pigeon Pose Arms Raised Chair

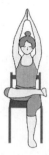

The Seated Pigeon Pose with Arms Raised Chair is a variation of the classic pigeon pose, designed for those who might find the traditional version a tad challenging or are in search of a seated alternative. In this adaptation, while seated comfortably in a chair, the practitioner places one ankle on the opposite thigh, creating a figure-four shape with the legs. This already gently opens the hip. To enhance the stretch and also involve the upper body, the arms are raised overhead. This movement stretches the hips and targets the upper back and the area between the shoulder blades.

The pose offers a dual advantage. First, it acts as a gentle hip opener, stretching the external hip muscles and relieving tightness in this area, often developed from prolonged sitting or standing. The positioning of the knee also imparts a subtle stretch to the quadriceps. Secondly, by raising the arms, there's an added benefit to the upper back, which can alleviate tension between the shoulder blades, a common area of tightness for many.

While generally safe, individuals with acute hip or knee injuries should approach this pose with caution. The elevation of the arms might not be suitable for those with specific shoulder or upper back issues. As with any yoga pose, it's essential to ensure comfort throughout the practice, making modifications as necessary. If any pain or discomfort arises, you should release the pose and consult a trained yoga instructor for guidance.

Steps (2 minutes)

1. Sit comfortably on a chair, ensuring both feet are flat on the ground.
2. Lift your right foot, placing the ankle on your left thigh, creating a figure four with your legs.
3. Ensure the right knee is pointing outwards, opening the hip.
4. Inhale deeply and, as you raise your arms, bring your palms together in front of your chest in Anjali Mudra (see p. 33), often associated with respect and balance.
5. Hold the position with your palms pressed together at your heart center, feeling the stretch in your hips and upper back for 1 minute.
6. Exhale, gently lowering your arms while maintaining the Anjali Mudra, and release your right foot back to the ground.
7. Repeat on the opposite side with the left foot on the right thigh, continuing to use the Anjali Mudra with your hands throughout the pose.

Bicep Curl Exercise Chair

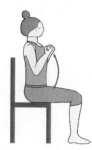

The Bicep Curl Exercise Chair is a revitalizing practice that infuses the body with energy. Designed as a preparatory movement, it sets the stage for more complex postures, blending seamlessly into various yoga flows. This exercise targets and strengthens the biceps at its heart, making it a key part of Chair Yoga and restorative sequences.

This pose primarily focuses on fortifying the biceps, offering toning and firming benefits. It also helps boost upper body endurance, aids in correcting posture, and enhances muscle coordination. Regular practice can lead to improved mobility and flexibility in the arms.

Although generally safe, those with recent arm, elbow, or shoulder injuries should proceed cautiously. It's always recommended to perform exercises within one's comfort zone, avoiding overextension or strain. If any discomfort arises, consulting with a qualified instructor or healthcare professional is advisable.

Steps (3 minutes)

1. Sit upright on a chair, with feet flat on the ground.
2. Clench your fists to form the Mushti Mudra (see p. 39). This involves curling your fingers into your palms and squeezing slightly, which can help release pent-up emotions or stress.
3. Keep your elbows close to your torso and ensure they are fully extended, maintaining the Mushti Mudra.
4. Inhale as you bend your elbows to bring your clenched fists towards your shoulders, emulating the curling motion.
5. Ensure the movement is isolated to your forearms while keeping the upper arms still.
6. Exhale while slowly lowering your clenched fists back to the starting position.
7. Repeat the movement for 3 minutes, maintaining the Mushti Mudra throughout the exercise.

Bound Hands Chair

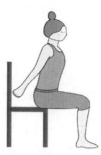

The Bound Hands Chair is a preparatory pose often used to warm up the body for more advanced yoga postures. Engaging the upper back muscles, this pose gently stretches and opens the shoulders, chest, and upper spine, proving particularly beneficial for those looking to alleviate tension in these areas.

The benefits of the Bound Hands Chair Pose are manifold. While it primarily focuses on the upper back, it also helps improve posture, enhance shoulder mobility, and promote relaxation. The gentle opening of the chest facilitates deeper breathing, which can be especially advantageous for those with respiratory issues.

However, it's essential to approach the Bound Hands Chair Pose with caution. Individuals with severe shoulder or upper back injuries should either avoid the pose or practice under the guidance of a certified instructor. Moreover, any sensation of pain or discomfort while in the posture is a signal to come out of it and seek modifications or alternatives. As always, listening to your body and adapting your practice according to your needs is essential.

Steps (2 minutes)

1. Settle into a chair with your feet planted firmly on the floor and your hips positioned a comfortable width apart.
2. Stretch your arms straight out in front of you, aligning them with your shoulders.
3. Cross your right arm over your left, bending both arms at the elbows.
4. Rotate your wrists and form the Vitarka Mudra (see p. 37) by touching the tips of your thumb and index finger, creating a circle, extending the other fingers, and keeping the other fingers extended.
5. While maintaining the Vitarka Mudra, bring the palms together as closely as possible, elevating the elbows slightly while keeping the shoulders relaxed.
6. Hold the position for 1 minute, feeling a stretch across the shoulders and upper back and experiencing the calmness brought by the Vitarka Mudra.
7. Release the arms and repeat on the opposite side, this time with the left arm over the right, continuing to hold the Vitarka Mudra.
8. After completing both sides, relax your arms by your sides and observe any sensations in the shoulders and upper back, maintaining a sense of truth and openness as symbolized by the Vitarka Mudra.

Cat Pose Variation Elbows

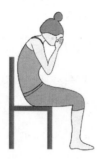

The Cat Pose Variation Elbow is a seated adaptation of the traditional Cat Pose, tailor-made for Chair Yoga. When practicing this pose, you mainly activate your core muscles, providing a gentle stretch and engagement of the abdominal area. This makes it a handy pose to include in sequences focusing on core strength.

Given its seated nature, this variation finds its place in Chair Yoga routines, offering accessibility to those who might find traditional floor-based poses a bit challenging. It's also featured in core-centric yoga sequences, emphasizing abdominal engagement and spine flexibility.

While the specific benefits of the Cat Pose Variation Elbow are not listed, one can infer from its traditional counterpart that it aids in improving posture, enhancing spine flexibility, and strengthening the abdominal muscles.

However, individuals with severe back issues or recent abdominal surgeries should approach this pose with caution. It's always advised to listen to your body and, if any discomfort arises, make the necessary adjustments or skip the pose. Consulting with a qualified yoga instructor is always beneficial, especially for those new to the practice or with underlying health concerns.

Steps (3 minutes)

1. Settle into a chair with your feet planted firmly on the floor and your hips positioned a comfortable width apart.
2. Certainly, here's how you could incorporate the Tattva Mudra (see p. 35) into the revised step.
3. Gently lift your hands to your face. As you support your head with your hands, form the Tattva Mudra by touching the tips of your thumbs to the tips of your ring fingers while keeping the other fingers extended. Ensure your neck is relaxed and your posture is maintained without strain. Inhale deeply, slightly arching your back and lifting your chest and chin towards the ceiling, keeping the Tattva Mudra.
4. While exhaling, curve your back, lower your chin toward your chest, and softly push your interlocked fingers in Tattva Mudra against your thighs.
5. Focus on engaging your core muscles, drawing your navel towards your spine during the exhale, and keeping the integrity of the Tattva Mudra.
6. Continue to flow between the arched and rounded positions, synchronizing with your breath and preserving the Tattva Mudra throughout.
7. Repeat this movement for 3 minutes, ensuring smooth transitions and deep breaths, all while maintaining the Tattva Mudra.

Cat Pose Variation

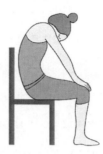

The Cat Pose Variation is a modified version of the traditional Seated Cat Pose, tailored for those seeking additional support. Practiced on a chair, it helps activate the muscles around the spine, promoting greater flexibility in the back, neck, and shoulders. This pose is a gateway to the Chair Cat-Cow Pose, and numerous other Chair Yoga flows. Stretching the entire back of the body it instills tranquility and composure. Such a pose turns out to be a refreshing break, especially in desk yoga routines, as it simultaneously eases physical and emotional tension. The forward bend incorporated in this pose gently compresses the abdomen, which may aid digestion. Its cooling and calming nature makes it a valuable addition to evening routines, particularly for those grappling with insomnia. Given the chair's support, it's an accessible option for the elder community.

Among the benefits of the Cat Pose Variation are its suitability for beginners due to its simplicity and the chair's stability. It's particularly advantageous for individuals who might experience dizziness or find the traditional Cat Pose challenging due to balance or strength issues. It's also helpful in therapeutic yoga, assisting those with knee problems, those recovering from herniated discs, or post-hip replacement surgery. The pose prevents stiffness for those confined to desks and benefits those with special needs, ensuring their muscles stay active and strong.

However, there are certain precautions to observe. For instance, individuals with recent surgeries or injuries related to the neck, spine, shoulders, or hips should practice cautiously and seek medical advice. Those with chronic back pain, heart conditions, high blood pressure, or severe digestive issues should approach this pose under expert guidance. Finally, choosing a chair is crucial to ensure safety and effectiveness in the pose.

Steps (3 minutes)

1. As you sit, place your hands in your lap in the Dhyana Mudra (see p. 40), with one hand on top of the other, palms facing upward. Gently touch your thumbs together, forming a subtle oval shape. This mudra fosters a sense of calm and meditation.

2. Focus on maintaining the Dhyana Mudra, which helps anchor your awareness and deepen your focus. As you breathe and move within the pose, let the mudra enhance your sense of inner peace.

3. With each exhale, gently accentuate the cat-like rounding of your spine, all while keeping your hands in the Dhyana Mudra. This combination allows for a continuous flow of energy and mindfulness throughout the pose.

4. Hold the Cat Pose Variation for 3 minutes, maintaining the Dhyana Mudra throughout. This steady mudra helps cultivate a meditative state even as you engage in the physical posture.

5. While in the Cat Pose Variation, emphasize breath awareness. The blend of gentle movement and the Dhyana Mudra aids in opening the upper back, shoulders, and neck, promoting a relaxed and positive energy flow.

Routine 2

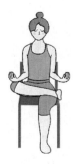 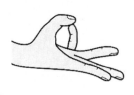

Sited Pigeon Pose Palms Up Chair with Jala Mudra
(2 minutes)

It is on a chair with feet grounded. Place the right ankle on the left thigh, gently pressing the right knee. Turn palms upward for an open chest. Breathe deeply, feeling the hip stretch. Hold this position for 1 minute, then switch sides and repeat for 1 minute.

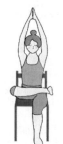 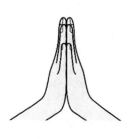

Seated Pigeon Pose Arms Raised Chair with Anjali Mudra
(2 minutes)

Sit on a chair with feet grounded. Place one ankle on the opposite thigh, opening the hip. Inhale, raising arms overhead. Feel the hip and upper back stretch. Exhale, lower arms. Hold this position for 1 minute, then switch sides and repeat for 1 minute.

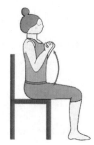 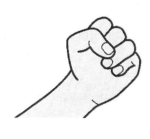

Bicep Curl Exercise Chair with Mushti Mudra
(3 minutes)

While seated upright on a chair, hold weights with palms forward. Curl weights towards shoulders, bending at the elbows, then slowly lowering them. Keep upper arms stationary and repeat for 3 minutes.

All pose images are copyright by Tummee - sequencing platform for yoga teachers

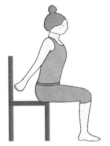 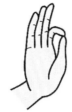

Bound Hands Chair with Vitarka Mudra
(2 minutes)

While seated with feet grounded, cross your arms, bending at the elbows. Rotate wrists to press palms together, elevating elbows slightly. Feel the stretch across the shoulders and upper back. Hold this position for 1 minute, then switch sides and repeat for 1 minute. Relax and observe sensations.

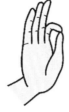

Cat Pose Variation Elbows with Tattva Mudra
(3 minutes)

Gently lift your hands to your face. Ensure your neck is relaxed and your posture is maintained without strain. Inhale deeply, slightly arching your back and lifting your chest and chin towards the ceiling. Hold this pose for 3 minutes.

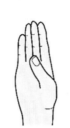 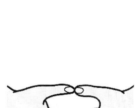

Cat Pose Variation with Dhyana Mudra
(3 minutes)

Settle into the chair. As you breathe deeply, gently round your spine with each exhale, maintaining the mudra to deepen focus and foster calm. Hold this pose for 3 minutes, allowing the combination of movement and mudra to open your upper back, shoulders, and neck, enhancing a sense of peace and relaxation.

Routine 3

Seated Forward Fold Pose Chair

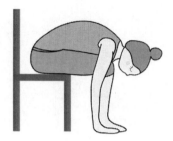

The Seated Forward Fold Pose Chair is exceptionally useful for individuals recovering from medical procedures or surgeries. It provides relief from tension built up due to prolonged desk work, targeting areas like the neck, shoulders, and lower back.

This pose specifically benefits the muscles of the lower back and gluteus.

This pose can significantly alleviate tension in the upper body. Although it mirrors the effects of the Standing Forward Fold Pose, the intensity of the hamstring and lower back stretch is lessened. This makes it an ideal pose for releasing muscle stiffness and tightness, particularly in the upper body. The pose is also beneficial for individuals recovering from trauma, as it promotes calmness and aids in combating insomnia. Long-haul travelers can use this pose to relieve the heaviness in the neck and shoulders. Furthermore, it aids in the healing process of various ailments and is a boon for older adults, especially those suffering from arthritis, osteoporosis, or tailbone pain.

Like all yoga poses, the Seated Forward Fold Pose Chair comes with its set of precautions. Those on blood pressure medication should be cautious, especially if they find breathing challenging during the pose. Individuals with Irritable Bowel Syndrome (IBS) should ensure they're comfortable, possibly using a cushion for added abdominal support. As always, personal comfort and safety should be of paramount importance.

Steps (3 minutes)

1. Begin by sitting comfortably in the Mountain Pose Chair (see p. 54), taking a moment to lengthen the spine and engage in several deep breaths. In this starting position, form the Tattva Mudra (see p. 35) by joining the tips of your thumb and index finger, creating a circle while keeping the other fingers straight. This mudra symbolizes truth and honesty.
2. With an inhalation, lengthen your torso upwards, maintaining the Tattva Mudra.
3. As you exhale, slowly lower your arms towards your feet while holding the Tattva Mudra.
4. Let your entire upper body rest on your thighs, positioning your chin near your knees and directing your gaze towards your feet.
5. Breathe deeply, gently pushing your torso closer to your thighs. If possible, lay your palms flat on the floor.
6. Stay in this position for 3 minutes, using each exhalation to move your chest and shoulders further from the thighs and deepen the forward bend.
7. To exit the pose, first, look up at an inhalation while releasing the Tattva Mudra. Then, lift your arms upwards and return to the seated Mountain Pose Chair position. If desired, take a moment to relax and repeat the sequence, extending the duration.

Seated Half Forward Fold Pose Chair

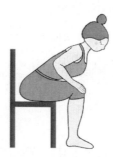

The Seated Half Forward Fold Pose Chair is a modified yoga pose specifically designed for Chair Yoga sequences. It targets the lower back, hips, pelvic region, and the psoas muscle, making it an effective addition to Chair Yoga routines.

This pose offers potential benefits for the areas it targets, although the specific benefits of the Seated Half Forward Fold Pose Chair are still being compiled. Once available, these details will provide a more in-depth understanding of the pose's impact on the body.

However, like any yoga pose, it's important to approach the Seated Half Forward Fold Pose Chair with caution. There may be contraindications associated with the pose that are yet to be detailed. As with any yoga practice, being aware of your body and any potential discomfort is vital. If you have specific health concerns, consulting with a professional before practicing is always a good idea.

Steps (3 minutes)

1. Begin by sitting upright in the Mountain Pose Chair (see p. 54).
2. Ensure your feet are firmly on the floor and aligned side by side.
3. Inhale deeply, lengthening your spine. As you do this, form the Vayu Mudra (see p. 36), by folding your index fingers so that they touch the base of your thumbs while extending the other fingers.
4. As you exhale, hinge at the hips and lean your torso forward to a comfortable halfway point, maintaining the Vayu Mudra with your hands.
5. Extend your arms forward, keeping them parallel to the ground or resting them on your thigh.
6. Keep your spine straight and gaze down, ensuring your neck is aligned with the spine.
7. Breathe deeply, feeling the stretch in your lower back and hips, and experiencing the calming effect of the Vayu Mudra. Hold this pose for 3 minutes.
8. To return, inhale and lift your torso back to the starting position, sitting upright.
9. Pause for a moment, feeling the effects of the stretch and the Vayu Mudra, before repeating or moving on to another pose.

Seated Forward Fold Pose Chair Variation Arm Crossed

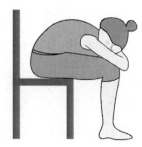

The Seated Forward Fold Pose Chair Variation with Arms Crossed is a modified version of the traditional seated forward fold, adapted to be performed on a chair. This pose offers a unique blend of stretches targeting several muscle groups.

In this variation, individuals sit on a chair and lean forward, crossing their arms as they do so. This position primarily targets the lower back, core, hips, neck, and pelvic muscles, providing a gentle yet effective stretch.

The pose is a staple in Chair Yoga sequences, often included in routines focusing on core and hip opening exercises. Its adaptability makes it a favorite among those who might find traditional floor-based poses challenging.

While specific benefits of this particular variation are yet to be listed, given the muscles it targets, one can infer that it aids in alleviating lower back tension, enhancing core strength, and promoting hip flexibility. The pose might also offer relief from neck strain and support pelvic muscle relaxation.

Although the pose is generally safe, those with specific health conditions or recent surgeries might need to approach it with caution. For instance, individuals with severe back or neck issues or certain abdominal conditions should seek advice from a medical professional or a trained yoga instructor before attempting the pose. As always, it's essential to prioritize comfort and avoid any position that induces pain.

Steps (3 minutes)

1. Sit upright on a chair, ensuring your feet are flat on the ground and spaced hip-width apart.
2. Lengthen your spine, taking a moment to breathe deeply.
3. As you breathe out, start to bend from your hips, tilting your upper body forward.
4. As you fold, cross your arms, forming the Mushti Mudra (see p. 39), by clenching your fists with your thumbs inside, letting them hang, or placing them on your thighs.
5. Ensure your spine remains elongated, avoiding any hunching while maintaining the Mushti Mudra.
6. Let your neck be an extension of your spine, gazing downward without straining and keeping your fists clenched in Mushti Mudra.
7. Feel the stretch across your lower back, hips, and the back of your thighs as the Mushti Mudra helps channel a release of pent-up emotions or tension.
8. Hold the pose for 3 minutes, tuning into the sensations in your body and the effect of the Mushti Mudra.
9. To come out, inhale and gently lift your torso, uncrossing your arms and releasing the Mushti Mudra, returning to an upright seated position.
10. Take a few breaths to settle and absorb the benefits of the stretch and the Mushti Mudra.

Head Up Chair

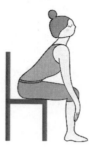

The Head Up Chair Pose is a therapeutic yoga position commonly included in Chair Yoga sequences. It's particularly beneficial for those seeking a gentler approach to yoga, such as prenatal participants or individuals engaged in restorative practices. By adopting this pose, practitioners can target specific muscle groups.

Although the precise benefits of the Head-Up Chair Pose are still being compiled, like many yoga poses, it likely offers a blend of relaxation, flexibility, and strength-building benefits. Additionally, this pose might be particularly helpful for those who spend extended periods sitting or working at desks, as it could aid in alleviating stress and tension.

However, as with any exercise, it's crucial to be aware of any contraindications. While specific considerations for the Head Up Chair Pose aren't provided at this moment, consulting a yoga instructor or healthcare professional is always advisable if you have underlying health concerns or conditions. It's essential to ensure that any yoga pose or exercise is safe and beneficial for your unique circumstances.

Steps (2 minutes)

1. Begin by sitting upright on a sturdy chair, placing your feet flat on the ground.
2. Ensure your feet are hip-width apart and your knees are aligned with your ankles.
3. Rest your hands gently on your thighs or beside you on the chair, forming the Vitarka Mudra (see p. 37), by touching the tips of your thumb and index finger, creating a circle, while extending the other fingers.
4. Take a deep breath in, focusing on your posture and grounding yourself.
5. As you exhale, maintain the upright position, ensuring your spine is elongated.
6. Tilt your head slightly upwards, gazing towards the ceiling without straining your neck.
7. Softly activate your core muscles to maintain your posture.
8. Inhale and exhale deeply and steadily, sustaining the pose for 2 minutes with your hands in the Vitarka Mudra.
9. Notice the mild stretching sensation in your neck and the engagement of the muscles in your upper back.
10. To release, return your gaze to a neutral forward position and take a few breaths, noticing the sensations from the pose and the calmness from the Vitarka Mudra.

Cobra Pose Chair

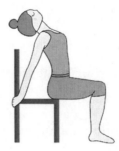

The Cobra Pose Chair is a modified version of the classic Cobra Pose, tailored for those who use a chair as a prop. This posture specifically targets and benefits the muscles of the mid-back, upper back, and chest, making it an excellent choice for individuals looking to enhance their spinal flexibility and strength.

Incorporated into various yoga sequences, the Cobra Pose Chair is often a key part of Chair Yoga routines and heart-opening sequences. This is because of its ability to expand the chest, promote better breathing, and foster a sense of openness in the heart region.

While the pose offers numerous advantages, it's essential to be mindful of certain precautions. Individuals with acute back or neck issues, or those who have recently undergone surgeries in these areas, should approach the Cobra Pose Chair with caution. It's recommended to seek guidance from trained yoga professionals. As always, practitioners should stay attuned to their body's signals and avoid any movements that result in discomfort.

Steps (2 minutes)

1. Sit relaxed at the center of the chair with your spine extended.
2. Reach behind to grasp the back of the chair with both hands, forming the Apana Mudra (see p. 41), by touching the tips of your thumb and middle finger while the other fingers remain extended.
3. Inhale and lift your chest and shoulders, directing your gaze upwards.
4. While exhaling, maintain the pose, feel the stretch in your neck and upper chest, and keep your hands in the Apana Mudra.
5. Hold this position, taking slow and deep breaths for 1 minute.
6. With every exhale, deepen the stretch and savor the sensation.
7. After 1 minute, release and return to a relaxed seated position.
8. Take a moment to absorb the feeling, then repeat the pose for another 1 minute, maintaining the Apana Mudra.
9. Recognize the rejuvenating energy flow in the throat area, which can help revitalize the voice and energy.

Cobra Pose Chair Variation Hands Chest

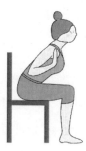

The Cobra Pose Chair with Hands Chest is a tailored variation of the traditional Cobra Pose, adapted for those who practice Chair Yoga. This version places a particular emphasis on activating and stretching specific muscles.

This pose is predominantly found in Chair Yoga sequences, catering to those who may find traditional mat yoga challenging or those seeking a quick stretch without leaving their chair.

While the specific benefits of this variation are still to be detailed, it likely offers some of the advantages of its traditional counterpart. These may include improved upper body flexibility, enhanced respiratory function due to the chest-opening nature of the pose, and a potential boost in mood from the gentle backbend.

However, as with all yoga poses, there are some precautions to consider. If you have any existing conditions or injuries, it's crucial to approach this pose cautiously. Specific contraindications for this variation haven't been provided, but it's always wise to consult with a yoga instructor or medical professional before adding new poses to your routine.

Steps (2 minutes)

1. Begin by sitting upright on a chair with your feet firmly planted on the ground.
2. Place your hands on the chest area, forming the Jala Mudra (see p. 42), by touching the tips of your thumb and little finger while the other fingers remain extended.
3. Take a deep breath, lengthening your spine.
4. As you exhale, gently lean back without straining, using your hands on your chest, maintaining the Jala Mudra, as support.
5. Keep your gaze forward or slightly upwards, ensuring you don't strain your neck.
6. Keep your shoulders relaxed and away from your ears.
7. Gently engage your core muscles to support the slight backbend.
8. Hold this position for 2 minutes, experiencing the stretch through your chest and upper back areas.
9. To come out of the pose, inhale and use your core strength to return to an upright seated position.
10. Rest for a moment, noticing the sensations in your body, then repeat if desired.

Routine 3

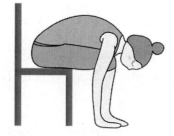 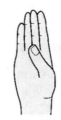

Seated Forward Fold Pose Chair with Tattva Mudra
(3 minutes)

Starting in the Mountain Pose Chair (see p. 54), inhale and extend your torso. As you exhale, lower your arms towards your feet. Rest torso on thighs with chin near knees. Deepen the bend with each breath, aiming for palms on the floor. After holding for 3 minutes, return to the starting position.

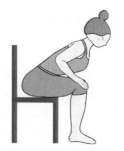 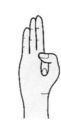

Seated Half Forward Fold Pose Chair with Vayu Mudra
(3 minutes)

Starting from the Mountain Pose Chair, practitioners lean forward while maintaining spinal alignment. Hold this pose for 3 minutes. This modification is especially beneficial for those with mobility limitations, allowing them to experience the stretch's benefits in a more accessible manner. After the pose, it's common to return upright and pause to internalize the effects.

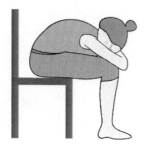 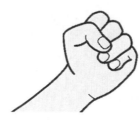

Seated Forward Fold Pose Chair Variation Arm Crossed with Mushti Mudra
(3 minutes)

While seated on a chair with feet flat and hip-width apart, inhale and lengthen the spine. Exhale, leaning forward from the hips and crossing your arms, either letting them hang or resting on your thighs. Maintain a straight spine and neutral neck, gazing downward. After holding for 3 minutes, return to an upright position, uncrossing the arms, and take a moment to relax and internalize the stretch's benefits.

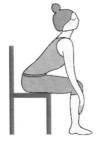 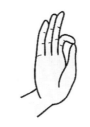

Head Up Chair with Vitarka Mudra
(2 minutes)

While seated on a chair with feet grounded, align your spine and tilt your head gently upwards, gazing at the ceiling. With hands resting on thighs and a deep, even breath, this pose helps activate the upper back muscles and offers a gentle neck stretch. After holding for 2 minutes, return to a neutral gaze and reflect on the sensations experienced.

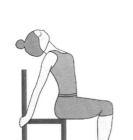 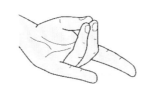

Cobra Pose Chair with Apana Mudra
(2 minutes)

Sit centered on a chair with a straight back. Grasp the chair's rear, inhale, and lift your chest, looking up. Exhale and savor the stretch in your neck and chest, holding for 1 minute. Release, rest, and repeat the pose for another 1 minute. This pose invigorates the throat, potentially restoring voice and energy.

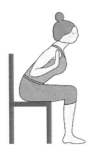 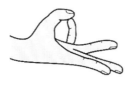

Cobra Pose Chair Variation Hands Chest with Jala Mudra
(2 minutes)

While seated upright in a chair, place your hands on your chest. As you breathe deeply, arch your back gently on the exhale, using your hands for support. Keep your gaze forward or tilt slightly upward without stressing the neck. Maintain relaxed shoulders and engage your core. After holding for 2 minutes, return to the starting position and relax before repeating.

Developing Core Strength and Flexibility

The Core Strength Importance for Mature Adults

As time marches on, aging inevitably brings a kaleidoscope of physiological changes our way. One of the most significant of these changes is in our muscular system. As we age, our muscles undergo atrophy, shrinking in size and weakening in strength. This isn't just a cosmetic concern; it profoundly impacts our mobility and overall quality of life.

The core, a complex network of muscles encircling our midsection, is arguably one of our body's most critical muscle groups. It's not all about flaunting a "six-pack" or looking good; the core is our body's powerhouse. It acts as a protective shield around our internal organs, supports the spine, and serves as a pivotal link connecting our upper and lower body.

Consider our everyday activities—bending to tie shoes, reaching up to grab something from a shelf, or even just sitting upright in a chair—all these actions call upon the core. For mature adults, who might already be grappling with challenges in routine tasks, the significance of core strength becomes even more pronounced.

A robust core is not just about easing day-to-day activities. It's instrumental in ensuring balance and stability. As the foundation for all movement, a strong core can significantly lower the risk of falls—a major concern for many older adults. Falls can lead to serious injuries, especially since bone density also tends to diminish with age.

Moreover, posture, often overlooked, is deeply intertwined with the core. With advancing years, there's a natural tendency to slouch or hunch, leading to spinal curvatures and related issues. A sturdy core aids in maintaining an erect and healthy posture, which promotes efficient breathing and organ function, and exudes confidence.

In the context of mature adults, it's not just about possessing core strength for strength's sake. It's about ensuring an independent, active, and fulfilling lifestyle. Simple pleasures, whether playing with grandchildren, gardening, or enjoying a leisurely walk, become more achievable and enjoyable with a strong and supple core.

In summary, while every muscle plays its part in our overall well-being, the core's importance is magnified as we age. It truly forms the epicenter of our physical function, ensuring we lead a life marked by activity, balance, and grace.

Understanding the Core

The term "core" often brings to mind images of chiseled abs, intense fitness routines, and perhaps even those enviable beach bodies. However, the true significance of the core runs much deeper and is more fundamental than these superficial associations.

Defining the Core Muscles

At its heart, the core is our body's central structure, the epicenter of balance, and the origin of most of our movements. Contrary to popular belief, the core goes beyond just the abdominal muscles. It's a complex web of muscles wrapping around our midsection, safeguarding our internal organs and spinal cord. The key players in this muscular network include:

- **Rectus Abdominis:** Commonly known as the "sixpack," this muscle is the most forward-facing of the abdominal muscles, running vertically along the front of the abdomen.
- **Obliques:** These are located on the sides of our midsection, responsible for the lateral bending and rotation of the trunk.
- **Transverse Abdominis**: This is the deepest layer, wrapping around the spine for protection and stability.
- **Erector Spinae:** A group of muscles running vertically along the spinal bones, crucial for keeping the back straight and rotating it.
- **Pelvic Floor Muscles:** These form the foundation of the core and play a vital role in supporting our internal organs and maintaining intra-abdominal pressure.

Role in Everyday Movement

The core's importance becomes clear when you consider that almost every action, whether as mundane as lifting a grocery bag or as intense as weightlifting at the gym, requires engagement. These muscles are the unsung heroes, providing stability, ensuring proper posture, and driving movement. They act as a bridge, transferring power between the upper and lower limbs, making sure our body functions as a cohesive unit.

For instance, when you turn to reach for something behind you, it's not just your arms at work. Your obliques and other core muscles are rotating the spine. When you stand up from a sitting position, the erector spinae contracts to straighten your back, while the rectus abdominis and transverse abdominis engage to stabilize the movement.

Moreover, a robust core is paramount for balance. Whether you're walking on an uneven path, standing in a moving bus, or practicing yoga, your core muscles are constantly adjusting and compensating to keep you upright and prevent falls.

In essence, understanding the core is about recognizing its central role in almost every aspect of our daily physical lives. From simple tasks to complex activities, the core is the unsung hero, ensuring efficiency, stability, and balance.

Benefits of a Strong Core

- **Back Pain Prevention:** One of the key benefits of having a strong core is a reduced susceptibility to back discomfort. The muscles in your core are essential for providing support to your spine. When these muscles are robust and efficient, they lighten the load on the spine, minimizing the risk of injuries and chronic back pain, a common issue among older adults.
- **Improved Balance and Stability:** Our core muscles are central to our ability to balance, a skill that becomes increasingly vital as we age. A strong core ensures that the body can maintain stability during movements and while stationary. It is especially crucial for older adults, as improved balance can significantly reduce the risk of falls, which can have serious consequences in later years.

- **Enhanced Posture:** Posture is about more than just standing up straight; it involves aligning the spine and reducing unnecessary strain on muscles and joints. A robust core facilitates better posture by ensuring the body maintains an upright and aligned position. This is particularly important for older adults, as the natural aging process can lead to spinal curvature, often resulting in posture-related ailments.
- **Better Respiratory Function:** The core's anatomy includes the diaphragm, a major muscle involved in breathing. When the core is strong, the diaphragm and surrounding muscles function more efficiently, allowing for deeper and more controlled breaths. It ensures that the respiratory system operates optimally, aiding overall health and well-being.

The Role of Flexibility

Strength and flexibility work together, shaping our physical capabilities. Strength anchors our body, providing the stability needed for daily activities, while flexibility ensures that our muscles and joints operate without restriction. Together, they form the foundation of our physical well-being. For example, a strong core is undoubtedly beneficial, but when paired with inflexible hip muscles, it can lead to alignment issues like anterior pelvic tilt, which may eventually manifest as back problems. As we age, our bodies transform. Muscles no longer stretch as they once did, and the range of movement in joints can decrease. Tendons and ligaments, vital connectors in our body, may become less supple. These changes can limit mobility and sometimes lead to discomfort. However, regular exercises aimed at enhancing flexibility can combat these natural aging progressions. Prioritizing flexibility ensures our joints remain fluid, movements stay graceful, and our range of motion persists without pain. As the golden years approach, maintaining flexibility becomes crucial for preserving our quality of life.

Chair Yoga's Approach to Core Strength and Flexibility

Chair Yoga offers a tailored approach to yoga, focusing on accessibility, especially for those who might find traditional yoga challenging. However, this adaptability doesn't mean it's any less effective in strengthening the core and enhancing flexibility. Many Chair Yoga poses actively engage the core muscles. Using the chair in various poses can sometimes add an extra layer of resistance, further intensifying the workout. Additionally, Chair Yoga provides a holistic exercise experience. Many of its poses, even if not specifically labeled as core or flexibility exercises, inherently serve these purposes. A prime example is maintaining an upright posture while seated without relying on the chair's backrest, activating the core muscles. This subtle engagement over time can significantly contribute to core strength and overall posture improvement.

Practicing Chair Yoga, particularly for older adults, requires a mindful approach. Practitioners must be attuned to their body's signals and understand its limits. Differentiating between productive stretching and potentially harmful discomfort is essential to avoid unnecessary stress or injury. Our body's recovery rate might not be as quick as we age, so caution is advised.

For older adults, diving into intense sessions occasionally might not be as beneficial as maintaining a steady, consistent routine. Gradual progression is key, allowing the body to adapt and grow stronger over time rather than being overwhelmed by sporadic bursts of strenuous activity.

Lastly, while Chair Yoga is designed for accessibility and safety, beginners, especially older individuals, should consider seeking advice from professionals. Engaging with a certified Chair Yoga instructor can be invaluable. They can offer insights into posture alignments, ensuring participants gain maximum benefits from each pose while minimizing any risk of injury. This guidance can serve as a foundation, allowing practitioners to engage in the practice more confidently and effectively in the long term.

Chapter 7: Chair Yoga for Upper and Lower Body Health

Targeting Neck, Shoulder, and Arm Strength

In this chapter, we delve into the specialized approach of Chair Yoga, focusing on the neck, shoulders, and arms. For many elders, the upper body often becomes a reservoir of stress and tension resulting from years of accumulated poor postural habits. It can lead to discomfort, reduced mobility, and sometimes even chronic pain.

Over prolonged periods, without proper ergonomic practices, many individuals develop a forward-leaning posture. This leaning, especially when spending hours over a desk or in sedentary activities, strains the neck and upper back muscles. Shoulders are not spared from the impact either; they begin to round forward, limiting their range of motion and strength.

But age doesn't only bring postural challenges. Natural conditions like osteoporosis can compromise bone strength, and the natural reduction in muscle mass can further intensify these challenges, making it even harder to maintain an upright posture or perform daily activities without some form of discomfort.

This is where Chair Yoga, with its adaptability and focus, offers an effective solution. It presents a series of poses designed specifically to combat the challenges faced by elders. These poses help in strengthening the muscles, compensating for the natural decline that comes with age. The emphasis on stretching in Chair Yoga enhances the elasticity of the muscles and tendons, which can significantly improve joint mobility. This is particularly beneficial for reducing the upper body's stiffness and tension.

Another important aspect of Chair Yoga is its focus on spinal alignment. The poses, even though performed while seated, emphasize maintaining a straight back, which in turn helps in correcting postural imbalances.

But the benefits aren't just physical. Incorporating mindful breathing and relaxation techniques in Chair Yoga helps alleviate pain and tension. Taking deep breaths improves blood circulation, supplying the muscles with the essential oxygen and nutrients they need.

On a broader spectrum, the practice of Chair Yoga also offers mental benefits. The emphasis on mindfulness helps reduce stress, brings mental clarity, and fosters a general sense of wellbeing.

In essence, Chair Yoga is a holistic practice tailored for elders, addressing both their physical and mental needs. Its regular practice can be the key to a more active, pain-free, and fulfilling life in the golden years.

The routines outlined in this chapter are crafted to cater to two core objectives.

Routine 1: Easing Tension in the Upper Body

Drawing from a variety of poses, this routine is thoughtfully designed to gently work through the layers of tension built up in the neck, shoulders, and arms. Through regular practice of these poses, students can hope to find relief from stiffness and discomfort, thereby promoting improved posture and overall well-being.

Routine 2: Exercises for Enhanced Posture

Postural integrity forms the cornerstone of overall physical health, especially as we age. This routine zeroes in on poses that not only strengthen the upper body but also aid in correcting and enhancing posture. It's a journey from understanding one's current postural habits to developing a more aligned, upright, and confident stance.

Each routine is designed to be 15 minutes long, featuring six poses. However, it is important to listen to your body. If you find it challenging to maintain a pose for the indicated time, do not worry. Hold each pose for as long as you feel comfortable, and with practice, you will gradually increase your endurance. There is no rush and no pressure—your comfort and safety are the most important.

Routine 1: Alleviating Tension and Pain in the Upper Body

Seated Shoulder Circles Chair

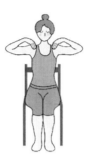

The Seated Shoulder Circles Chair is a fundamental warm-up movement, perfect for beginners, focusing mainly on the shoulders and upper back. Although it's a basic move, those suffering from shoulder and upper back stiffness may find it challenging initially. However, consistent practice can greatly increase joint mobility and strengthen the shoulders and arms.

This pose has versatile applications. While it can be performed standing, the seated version is specially designed for older adults or individuals with limited mobility. Its therapeutic attributes make it a beneficial component of recovery yoga, helping people regain mobility and strength after an injury. It's also an excellent quick remedy for tired shoulders and neck from daily activities and is a great addition to desk yoga routines.

Focusing on its benefits, the Seated Shoulder Circles Chair warms the body and prepares it for more demanding yoga poses or sequences. The movement strengthens the Rotator Cuff, fortifying the shoulder joint, which is essential for poses that demand shoulder strength, like arm balances and inversions.

Moreover, this movement encourages deeper breathing due to chest expansion, revitalizing both the brain and body. It also benefits senior yoga, relieving age-related conditions such as osteoporosis.

However, while it's predominantly safe, those with shoulder injuries should proceed cautiously. It's advisable to avoid the movement until fully healed. Those recovering from surgeries, especially around the heart, should also be cautious. Specific shoulder conditions might require a more cautious approach, but one can find relief from pain and stiffness with consistent practice.

Steps (2 minutes)

1. Begin in the Mountain Pose Chair (see p. 54). Sit with your spine erect and straight, grounding your sit bones firmly on the chair to relieve sacrum pressure. Roll your shoulders back and let them drop to avoid hunching.
2. Form the Mushti Mudra (see p. 39) by clenching your hands into fists. This mudra is known to release pent-up emotions and tension. Gently rest your clenched fists on your shoulders with your elbows bent.
3. As you inhale, raise your arms, allowing your elbows to point upwards, keeping the fists on your shoulders. Keep your arms close to your ears to maximize the shoulder joint's range of motion.
4. Continue inhaling, moving your bent arms backward, and feeling the expansion of the chest and diaphragm. This movement initiates the external rotation of the shoulder joint.
5. Begin to exhale, slowly lowering your arms until your elbows are beside your torso, maintaining the Mushti Mudra. As you exhale, bring your elbows in front of your chest, aiming to touch them together, or as close as comfort allows.
6. Perform these shoulder rolls for 1 minute, focusing on relaxed and regular breathing. The Mushti Mudra adds an element of focus and helps in releasing tension. Keep your neck relaxed throughout the movement.

7. After completing 1 minute, lower your arms and relax, releasing the Mushti Mudra. Pause to observe the sensations in your body and shoulders.
8. Repeat the circular motion in the opposite direction, re-forming the Mushti Mudra. Inhale as you open your elbows downward by your ribs, move them backward, then upwards, and exhale as you bring them forward.
9. Complete the shoulder rolls in this reverse direction for 1 minute.
10. Conclude the exercise by bringing your arms down by your sides, relaxing your hands, and releasing the Mushti Mudra. Take a few deep breaths, observing the effects of the practice on your shoulders and overall posture before transitioning to the next posture.

Hands Up Chair

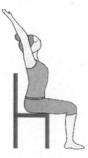

The Hands Up Chair pose is a vital element in various yoga sequences, especially for its profound impact on several muscle groups. Primarily targeting the arms, shoulders, and chest, it serves as a holistic exercise for the upper body. Its adaptability makes it suitable for various yoga styles. For instance, Chair Yoga sequences offer those with limited mobility the chance to experience the pose's benefits. In restorative yoga sequences, the pose acts as a soothing movement, aiding in relaxation and recovery. Moreover, it's significant in heart-opening yoga sequences, promoting chest expansion and deeper breathing.

While the benefits of the "Hands Up Chair" pose are numerous, they have yet to be documented in detail. Similarly, while yoga is generally safe, particular precautions should be considered when engaging in this pose, which also requires detailed analysis. Practitioners are always advised to listen to their bodies and seek guidance when uncertain.

Steps (2 minutes)

1. Sit comfortably, relax after the chest expansion pose, and take a few deep breaths.
2. Inhale deeply, lifting your arms above your head, which opens the chest and provides a full stretch to the shoulders and arms.
3. Incorporate the Jala Mudra (see p. 42), by forming a circle with the thumb and index finger while extending the other fingers to enhance focus and calm during the pose.
4. Exhale once you've raised your arms, maintaining the pose for 2 minutes, or as long as it feels comfortable.
5. If lifting both arms simultaneously is challenging, consider lifting one arm at a time or raising both arms as far as they'll go, even if it means having bent elbows.
6. The upward motion of the arms enhances heart function, aiding in better blood circulation and heart health.
7. Optionally close your eyes, tune into your inner self, and listen to the muffled sounds around you as your arms might partially block your ears.

Seated Twists Chair

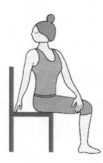

Seated Twists Chair, often incorporated in Chair Yoga sequences, offers a dynamic twist for the spine, upper back, hips, neck, and arms. Typically seen as a warm-up flow, this twist greatly enhances the flexibility of the spine, shoulders, and hips, keeping the joints active. It's particularly beneficial in senior yoga for its gentle yet effective movement.

This twist acts as a protective approach to address the neck, hips, and shoulders while working on the back muscles. The foundation of the movement is in extending and twisting, anchored by the sit bones on the chair. Regular practice maintains the spine's normal range of motion. Seated Twists Chair are invaluable for individuals who can't stand for extended periods during yoga sessions or find floor sitting challenging. Given its therapeutic nature, the practice benefits specific conditions like injury recovery, post-surgery rehabilitation, age-related constraints, body structure, and mental health. The chair's support allows for longer torso twists, ensuring breathwork aligns with body movement. Over time, it improves the spinal range of motion, leading to deeper twists.

Anatomically, Seated Twists Chair targets muscles like the arms, shoulders, lower, middle, and upper back, hips, and neck. They are commonly found in Chair Yoga, prenatal yoga, restorative yoga, and hip-opening yoga sequences.

The benefits of the Seated Twists Chair are multifaceted. They stretch the sides of the spine, with one side contracting and the other stretching, helping to alleviate mild back pain from prolonged sitting or age-related factors. The pose also enhances blood flow to the arms, shoulders, and neck, offering relief from muscle knots. It assists in detoxification, promoting prana or life force, leading to rejuvenation and stress relief. This twist also stimulates deeper breathing, ensuring efficient lung function, making it ideal for senior yoga sequences. The pose can be incorporated into therapeutic yoga, benefiting individuals with special needs or recovering from surgeries.

However, like all exercises, certain contraindications need consideration. Individuals with injuries or surgeries involving abdominal organs, pelvic floor, lower back, neck, shoulders, or spine should approach this pose with caution. Specific conditions like high blood pressure, heart problems, severe digestive disorders, or spinal issues like scoliosis require extra care. It's also essential to ensure the twist originates from the spine's base, not just the chest and shoulders.

Steps (2 minutes)

1. Sit comfortably on a chair, ensuring your back is straight. Place feet and knees about hip-width apart. Place your hands on your knees in Tattva Mudra (see p. 35), gently touching the tips of your thumb and index finger while keeping the other fingers extended. This gesture promotes truthfulness and clarity. Take a few deep breaths in this position.

2. Take a full breath in, lengthening your spine towards the ceiling as you press your sitting bones down into the chair, establishing a stable base for your posture. Maintain the Tattva Mudra to enhance your focus and breathing.

3. As you exhale, begin a twist to your right. Release the Tattva Mudra, placing your right hand on the back of the chair and your left hand outside your right thigh for support in the twist.

4. As you deepen the twist, ensure your left hip and thigh stay in place. Keep both

knees aligned, preventing the left knee from moving forward. Feel the twist along your spine.

5. Turn your head and set your gaze over your right shoulder, holding this position for 1 minute. The twist should be comfortable and without strain.
6. On an inhalation, release the twist and return to the center. Reestablish the Tattva Mudra on your knees, allowing a moment to re-center yourself.
7. Exhale and gently repeat the twist on the left side, ensuring a balanced approach on both sides. Hold this position for 1 minute.
8. Repeat the pose for several rounds, holding each side for a few seconds or continuous breaths, according to your comfort level. Remember to reengage the Tattva Mudra on your knees when you return to the center.

Goddess Pose On Chair

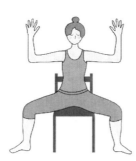

In the Seated Goddess Pose on the Chair, both the upper and lower body are actively engaged. When you raise your arms and elongate your spine, muscle groups like the glutes, quadriceps, inner thighs, hip flexors, and joints of the knees, hips, and feet become notably engaged and active.

The upper body experience in the Seated Goddess Pose on the Chair offers an advantage: the pose can be held longer as the hips and sit bones receive support and stability. This modified pose is beneficial for those facing challenges practicing on the mat due to physical conditions, age, or recovery from ailments or surgery. It can be practiced by anyone, making it suitable for corporate yoga sessions. This pose can be therapeutic as a gentle shoulder opener, addressing issues such as frozen shoulder, neck or shoulder tightness, or shallow breathing.

Anatomically, the Seated Goddess Pose on the Chair positively influences various muscles like the arms, shoulders, biceps, triceps, hips, knees, and pelvic region. Due to its structure and benefits, it's a common feature in Chair Yoga sequences, prenatal yoga sessions, and hip-opening yoga flows.

When discussing the benefits of the Goddess Pose On Chair, it's essential to recognize its dual foundation, incorporating elements of the Goddess Pose with Arms Down (see p. 159). This combination offers stability to both the upper and lower body, with engaged muscles gently stretching and contracting. It's particularly useful for students recovering from abdominal surgeries, providing a gentle stretch to the side back, rib cage, and abdominal muscles. Similarly, individuals recuperating from heart or spine surgeries can approach this variant with care, gradually extending the arms to improve breathing and reduce postoperative weakness. The flexed arms in this pose can also gently activate back muscles after spine surgery. With its therapeutic qualities, this pose can address numerous physical conditions, allowing yoga instructors to adapt it to the specific needs of their students.

Steps (3 minutes)

1. Begin by sitting comfortably on a chair, ensuring your back is straight. Place your feet and knees about hip-width apart and take a few deep breaths to center yourself.
2. Inhale deeply, extending your spine upwards while firmly grounding your sit bones on the chair, creating a solid foundation for your posture.
3. During the exhale, softly tilt forward from your waist. It's crucial to keep your spine long and straight, avoiding any slumping or rounding of the back.
4. With your hands on your waist, check that your knees are aligned with your ankles. Make any necessary adjustments to ensure proper alignment and balance.
5. Press firmly into all four corners of your feet, making sure that the outer edges of your feet remain grounded. Simultaneously, lift and energize the inner arches of your feet to prevent the knees from collapsing inward, promoting stability in the pose.
6. On your next inhalation, open your arms into a cactus position. It involves bending your elbows to form an L-shape at shoulder level, with your palms facing forward. As you do this movement, adopt the Vitarka Mudra (see p. 37), by touching the tips of your thumbs and index fingers, forming circles, while extending the other fingers. This mudra is known for enhancing communication and understanding.
7. Hold this position for 3 minutes. Focus on maintaining a straight spine and a forward gaze while keeping your shoulders relaxed and drawn back. The Vitarka Mudra aids in maintaining focus and clarity during this pose.

8. To release from the pose, exhale and gently place your hands back on your waist. Inhale deeply as you straighten your spine and adjust your feet back to their starting position, preparing to transition out of the pose.
9. Relax and take a few breaths, feeling the effects of the pose wash over you. Notice your body's balance of energy and relaxation, and appreciate the moment of peace you've created.

Seated Cactus Arms Chair

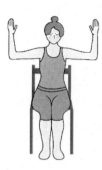

In The Seated Cactus Arms Chair pose, individuals sit upright on a chair, feet firmly grounded, as they open their arms out in a cactus shape, forming an L-shape at the sides. Tailored for those who might struggle with the traditional cross-legged position, this pose provides a comfortable alternative for beginners, individuals recovering from illnesses or injuries, or those with limited mobility.

This chair-based adaptation is versatile, making it suitable for a wide range of students and elderly categories. It's even applicable for desk-bound professionals, introducing a touch of 'Desktop Yoga' into their routine.

In the Seated Cactus Arms Chair pose, the chair's support allows the pose to be held for extended periods. This prolonged hold, combined with the open cactus arm position, can improve respiratory patterns and benefit those with respiratory conditions like asthma. Moreover, it strengthens the muscles of the chest, neck, arms, shoulders, and upper back. It can be particularly helpful in addressing postural issues such as a sunken chest or hunchback (kyphosis).

Incorporating this pose into restorative yoga sequences can relieve neck and shoulder tension, potentially aiding conditions like fibromyalgia and osteoporosis, and improving posture, balance, and overall strength.

The pose aids in opening the heart, which can be therapeutic for individuals with respiratory disorders. It's a versatile pose that can be introduced in various settings, from therapeutic sessions for individuals with special needs to regular yoga classes for working professionals or students. Importantly, those unable to sit on the floor due to conditions like knee arthritis can still engage in this variation. However, there are precautions to note. Be mindful of any existing injuries or recent surgeries related to your shoulders, spine, or arms that this pose might aggravate. It's also essential to approach the pose with gentleness, especially if it's part of a rehabilitation process after surgery.

Steps (3 minutes)

1. Ensure you have a suitable chair where your feet can comfortably touch the ground.
2. Sit upright in the Mountain Pose Chair (see p. 54): feet flat and together, knees over ankles, spine straight, chin level with the floor. Rest your arms on your knees with your hands in the Vayu Mudra (see p. 36), where the index finger folds to touch the base of the thumb, and the thumb gently presses on the index finger, while the other fingers remain extended.
3. Ground yourself by pressing your sit bones into the chair and taking a few deep breaths.
4. Inhale and extend your arms out to the sides at shoulder level.
5. As you exhale, bend your elbows, forming a cactus shape with your arms, creating an L-shape at your sides.
6. Keep your elbows aligned with your shoulders and palms facing forward. Here, the transition from Vayu Mudra to open palms with fingers spread wide and pointing upwards.
7. Hold the pose, feeling a stretch across your chest, for 3 minutes.
8. As you inhale, expand your chest and draw your shoulder blades together. On the exhale, engage your biceps and triceps, imagining you're pushing your forearms backward without actually moving them.
9. Exhale and lower your arms to rest on your knees, returning to the Mountain Pose Chair with your hands back in the Vayu Mudra.

Mountain Pose Raised Hands Chair

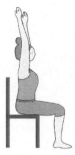

In The Mountain Pose with Raised Hands, practitioners enjoy an accessible stretch for the arms, shoulders, chest, and back, making it particularly beneficial for beginners, mature adults, or those with certain physical limitations.

Being seated provides an opportunity for those who might find it challenging to stand for extended periods or to sit on the floor. This pose strengthens the upper body, fostering a sense of lightness and expansiveness, particularly valuable for those recovering from surgeries or medical treatments. By emphasizing proper posture, this pose aims to alleviate tension commonly found in the neck, shoulders, and back, a frequent issue arising from modern sedentary lifestyles.

When executed, the pose encourages the practitioner to sit upright on a chair, extending their arms skyward. It not only stretches the arms and shoulders but also aids in opening the chest. This action can improve breathing and introduce a calming effect, which is especially beneficial for individuals with respiratory challenges. Furthermore, stretching the abdominal region can also stimulate the digestive system.

However, the pose is not without its precautions. Those with recent injuries or surgeries should approach the pose cautiously and under expert guidance, particularly in the neck, arms, or back regions. It's essential to ensure the chosen chair provides adequate support. While straightforward, the pose requires careful attention to one's body, ensuring alignment and avoiding overstretching. Additionally, individuals with conditions like high or low blood pressure or those with a history of cardiac issues should practice with awareness. For those experiencing tailbone pain or lower back issues, using a cushioned chair or additional support might be beneficial.

In essence, the Mountain Pose with Raised Hands is versatile and inclusive, acting as a therapeutic and strengthening exercise, easily adapted to various needs and circumstances. Its emphasis on posture and alignment makes it an ideal antidote to the strains of modern life, offering a moment of grounding and relaxation.

Steps (3 minutes)

1. Sit upright on a chair, ensuring your spine is straight. Place your feet and knees about hip-width apart, and take a few calming breaths, grounding yourself on the chair.
2. Position your feet parallel to each other, maintaining a small distance between them. Breathe deeply and relax for 2–3 breaths.
3. Inhale and extend your arms overhead, keeping them parallel to one another. As you do this movement, form the Lotus Mudra (see p. 38), by bringing your palms together, keeping the base of the palms, little fingers, and thumbs touching while spreading the other fingers apart like the petals of a lotus flower.
4. Maintain an upright posture with a straight back, holding the pose for 3 minutes while focusing your gaze forward.
5. Exhale and slowly bring your arms down to return to the initial seated position.

Routine 1: Alleviating Tension and Pain in the Upper Body

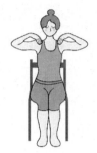 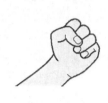

Seated Shoulder Circles Chair with Mushti Mudra
(2 minutes)

Sit upright in the Mountain Pose Chair (see p. 54), with fingertips touching the shoulders. Try to touch bent elbows in front. While inhaling, raise your arms, pointing elbows upward, then move them backward. On an exhale, lower the elbows to your sides and then bring them forward. Continue this motion for 1 minute, then relax. Reverse the direction for another 1 minute and conclude by resting your arms at your sides.

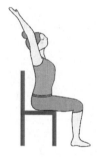 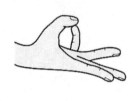

Hands Up Chair with Jala Mudra
(2 minutes)

Begin seated comfortably. Inhale deeply, lifting your arms overhead, stretching both shoulders and expanding the chest. If lifting both arms is challenging, modify them by raising them one at a time or with a slight bend at the elbows. Hold this pose for 2 minutes. By closing your eyes, you can tune into your inner sounds for a moment of reflection.

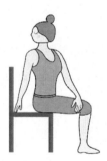 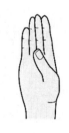

Seated Twists Chair with Tattva Mudra
(2 minutes)

Sit straight on a chair with feet hip-width apart. Inhale, elongating your spine. Exhale and twist to the right, placing your right hand behind you and your left hand on your right thigh. Ensure your knees stay aligned. Hold your gaze over the right shoulder for 1 minutes. Inhale back to center, then repeat on the left for 1 minute. Finish with gentle neck stretches.

All pose images are copyright by Tummee - sequencing platform for yoga teachers

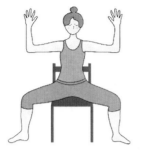 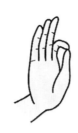

Goddess Pose On Chair with Vitarka Mudra
(3 minutes)

Spread your feet wider than your hips and angle your toes outward. With hands on your waist and a straight spine, inhale deeply, engaging your core. As you exhale, lean forward slightly. Align your knees with your ankles, grounding your feet firmly. Upon inhaling once more, stretch your arms into a cactus-like shape with your palms facing forward. Hold this position, gazing ahead with relaxed shoulders, for 3 minutes. Finally, exhale, return to the starting position, and relax, absorbing the benefits of the pose.

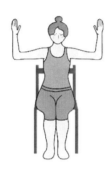 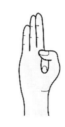

Seated Cactus Arms Chair with Vayu Mudra
(3 minutes)

Sit upright with your feet flat, establishing a strong foundation. Inhale, lifting your arms to shoulder level, and as you exhale, bend your elbows into a cactus shape. Maintain this position. Deepen the pose for 3 minutes, expanding your chest and engaging your arm muscles. Return your arms to the center and then lower them to your knees. Conclude by relaxing and focusing on deep, rhythmic breathing.

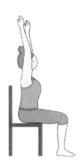 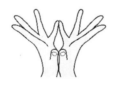

Mountain Pose Raised Hands Chair with Lotus Mudra
(3 minutes)

Sit on a chair and position your feet hip-width apart. Take a few grounding breaths, feeling the stability of your seat. Inhale and lift your arms overhead, ensuring they remain parallel to each other. Hold this extended posture for 3 minutes, gazing forward, and breathe deeply. Exhale, gently lowering your arms back to your sides. Conclude by relaxing and engaging in deep, rhythmic breathing.

Routine 2: Exercises for Enhanced Posture

Neck Rolls Chair A-B-C

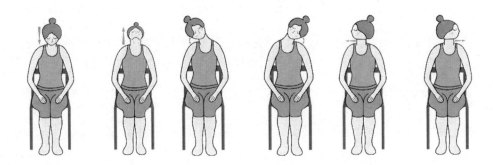

The Neck Rolls Chair series, encompassing variations A, B, and C, is a holistic approach to nurturing neck health and flexibility. It series of gentle yet effective exercises is designed to be performed while seated, making it an ideal routine for individuals of all ages and abilities, especially those with limited mobility or recovering from injuries.

Key Benefits of Neck Rolls Chair

- **Enhanced mobility:** Each variation targets different cervical spine movements, collectively enhancing the overall range of motion in the neck. This series addresses flexion, extension, lateral flexion, and rotation, ensuring a well-rounded approach to neck mobility.

- **Relief from stiffness:** Regular practice of these exercises can significantly alleviate stiffness and discomfort in the neck region. By gently stretching and mobilizing the neck muscles and joints, these exercises can help reduce the tension built up from routine activities or extended periods of sitting.

- **Improved posture:** As these exercises encourage the proper alignment and movement of the neck, they indirectly contribute to better posture. A mobile and flexible neck can lead to a more balanced and aligned posture, reducing strain on other parts of the
- spine.

Accessibility and Safety

Designed to be performed in a seated position using a chair for support, the Neck Rolls Chair series is accessible to those who may find standing exercises challenging. This added support provides stability, making it a safe option for seniors, office workers, or anyone needing a gentle yet effective neck workout.

Versatility in Practice

The Neck Rolls Chair series can be seamlessly integrated into various routines, whether as a warm-up in a yoga session, a midday break at the office, or part of a therapeutic regimen. Its adaptability ensures that it can be practiced almost anywhere—at home, at work, or even in a seated position during travel.

In conclusion, the Neck Rolls Chair series is a comprehensive solution for maintaining neck health and flexibility. With its focus on varied movements and ease of practice, it stands out as a valuable tool in anyone's wellness routine, promoting neck health, comfort, and overall wellbeing.

Steps (3 minutes)

1. **Start Position:** Start by sitting in a relaxed position on a chair, ensuring your feet are flat on the ground. Rest your hands gently on your thighs, palms facing upwards, and lightly touch the tips of your thumbs together to form the Dhyana Mudra (see p. 40). Take a moment to center yourself by taking a few deep breaths.

2. **Chair Neck Roll A (Flexion and Extension):**
   - Gradually bring your chin down towards your chest, experiencing a mild stretch along the back of your neck.
   - Maintain this posture briefly, then gently tilt your head backward, raising your chin towards the ceiling. This action provides a stretch to the front of your neck.

- Repeat these movements slowly, moving your head forward and backward, synchronizing with your breath. Do the movements for 1 minute.

3. **Chair Neck Roll B (Lateral Flexion):**
   - Return your head to a neutral position.
   - Carefully incline your head to the right, guiding your right ear closer to your right shoulder. Make sure not to elevate your shoulder to meet your ear.
   - Hold for a breath, then gently tilt your head to the left side.
   - Alternate between the right and left sides, doing this lateral flexion for 30 seconds on each side.

4. **Chair Neck Roll C (Rotation/Twisting):**
   - Again, start with your head in a neutral position.
   - Slowly turn your head to the right, aiming to look over your right shoulder. Ensure your shoulders remain relaxed and facing forward.
   - Hold for a breath, then gently turn your head to the left, attempting to look over your left shoulder.
   - Continue alternating this neck rotation for 30 seconds on each side.

5. **Completion:**
   - Once you've completed all cycles, bring your head back to the neutral position.
   - Take a few deep breaths, feeling the release of tension in the neck and upper back areas.

This sequence of Neck Rolls Chair A, B, and C effectively warms up the neck, increasing the range of motion and preparing the body for more intense yoga poses or flows. These movements target critical areas around the cervical spine, promoting flexibility, relieving tension, and enhancing overall neck health. Remember to execute these exercises with gentleness and stay within your comfort zone to avoid any potential strain.

Neck Stretch Chair

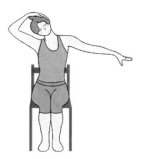

The Neck Stretch Chair primarily serves as a warm-up. This seated exercise illuminates the entire spine and helps alleviate shoulder, neck, and upper back tension. As you roll your shoulders back and open your chest to do it, you can destress and unwind. Its safety is its most significant advantage, making it accessible and risk-free for everyone.

This neck elongation is a staple in Yoga for the Golden-Agers. Its gentle synchronization of breath with movement makes it a perfect fit for Restorative flows or Postnatal Yoga, especially when the Standing Neck Stretch feels a bit too challenging.

From an anatomical standpoint, the Neck Stretch Chair predominantly targets the neck muscles. It prepares the body, gearing it up for more intensive yoga postures or flows.

However, if there are any specific contraindications associated with the Neck Stretch Chair, you're advised to consult with a professional or check back here for updates.

Steps (2 minutes)

1. Find a comfortable seated position on your chair, with both feet flat on the ground. Allow your hands to rest effortlessly by your sides. Close your eyes for a moment and focus on your breath, grounding yourself in the present.
2. With a deep inhalation, prepare to engage the Apana Mudra (see p. 41), with your left hand by bringing the tips of the thumb, middle finger, and ring finger together, and extending the other fingers. This mudra supports the body's natural detoxification processes. Keep your right hand free, as it will be used to assist in the neck stretch.
3. As you continue to breathe deeply, gently use your right hand to guide your head to the right, feeling a stretch along the left side of your neck. Simultaneously, maintain the Apana Mudra with your left hand held at your side or in your lap, whichever feels more comfortable and balanced.
4. Hold the stretch for 1 minute, savoring the extension along your neck. Allow the Apana Mudra to contribute to a sense of release and purification as you maintain your position.
5. On an inhalation, carefully bring your head back to a neutral position, releasing the guidance of your right hand. As you exhale, relax both your arms back to your sides and release the Apana Mudra with your left hand.
6. Repeat the neck stretch on the opposite side, holding the stretch for 1 minute, always using the opposite hand to perform the mudra. Throughout this practice, stay mindful of your core engagement, which supports your posture and enhances the exercise's benefits to your body's alignment and internal balance.

Seated Side Stretch Pose Chair

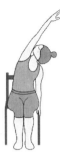

The Seated Side Stretch Pose Chair is a clever adaptation of traditional yoga poses, utilizing a chair for support to make it accessible to a wider array of individuals. In this practice, while seated, one extends an arm across to the opposite side, forming a gentle curve in the spine. This asymmetrical pose actively engages torso muscles, including the shoulders, upper back, chest, and even parts of the core and psoas.

This pose is therapeutic. It's especially beneficial for those recovering from surgeries or medical treatments like chemotherapy or those who find it challenging to stand for extended periods. Moreover, this pose can counteract the hours many spend hunched over computer screens by releasing accumulated tension, thus promoting relaxation in the neck, back, and shoulders.

Due to its gentle nature, this pose can be included in routines designed for mature adults or those in need of restorative yoga. One of its primary benefits is the opening of the shoulders, optimizing diaphragm function, which can be particularly helpful for those with respiratory issues like asthma.

Anatomically, this pose targets various muscles, notably in the arms, shoulders, upper back, chest, and neck. Its stretching effect aids in lengthening and relaxing these muscle groups. The chair serves not just as a support but also enhances the range of motion during the stretch, making it more effective and comfortable, especially for beginners or those with limited mobility.

However, while the Seated Side Stretch Pose Chair is generally safe, those with injuries in the arms, shoulders, neck, ribcage, or spine or who have undergone abdominal surgeries should approach this pose cautiously and preferably under expert guidance. Also, those with conditions like high or low blood pressure or vertigo should consult with a knowledgeable yoga instructor. Lastly, the choice of chair is crucial. It's best to opt for one with a back and, ideally, without armrests to ensure safety and maximize the pose's benefits.

Steps (2 minutes)

1. Begin by sitting comfortably, hands resting by your side, and close your eyes. Take a few deep breaths to center yourself. As you do this, form the Mushti Mudra (see p. 39), by curling your fingers into fists, thumbs resting on top of the fingers.
2. Inhale, lifting your right arm upward, maintaining the Mushti Mudra. While doing this, softly tilt your upper body and neck to the left, creating a stretch along the right side of your body.
3. Exhale completely while holding the stretch, feeling the expansion on your right side. Breathe here for 1 minute, keeping your right hand in the Mushti Mudra.
4. On your next inhale, straighten and extend your right arm with the Mushti Mudra, then slowly lower it back to the chair as you exhale.
5. Repeat the same movement with your left arm, ensuring you maintain balance and don't lean too far to the left. Form the Mushti Mudra with your left hand as well. Hold this stretch for 1 minute.
6. Remember to engage your core and maintain stability throughout the stretch, keeping the Mushti Mudra in both hands to enhance focus and energy.

Seated Cactus Arms Together Chair

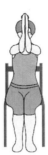

The Seated Cactus Arms Together Chair pose is a shoulder movement characterized by shoulder abduction, where they move away from each other, providing a deep muscle stretch. This pose can be approached in various ways:

- As a dynamic movement, it serves as a warm-up for the shoulders and arms, enhancing their range of motion.
- It's beneficial for individuals undergoing rehabilitation post-shoulder injury or surgery, though they must practice under a yoga teacher's guidance.
- This pose can alleviate shoulder stiffness and tightness for those spending prolonged periods at a desk.
- Older adults can also adopt this practice to relieve tension in the upper body.

This pose acts as a preparatory step for more rigorous yoga poses or flows, focusing attention on the arms and shoulders. As for its benefits, while the specifics are still being compiled, the pose is known to ease tension and improve shoulder mobility.

When practicing this pose, older adults and those with shoulder conditions or post-surgery need to seek professional guidance to avoid strain. Heart patients, especially post-surgery, should consult their doctor before attempting it. Proper breathing is crucial due to the pose's compressive nature on the upper body.

Steps (3 minutes)

1. Start by sitting comfortably in your chair, taking a moment to become present with your breath.
2. As you breathe in, lift your arms to shoulder height, bending your elbows with your palms facing each other.
3. Exhale and spread your fingers wide, transitioning into the Lotus Mudra (see p. 38), by bringing the bases of your palms and tips of your fingers together while allowing the other parts of your fingers to open gently, resembling the petals of a lotus flower.
4. On your next inhalation, while maintaining the Lotus Mudra, slowly bring your arms forward, feeling the expansion across your chest.
5. Hold the Lotus Mudra and the closed arm position for 3 minutes as you exhale, noticing the sensations in your hands, arms, and chest.
6. Continue this movement, coordinating your breath with the opening and closing of the Lotus Mudra, for three complete cycles.
7. Upon completing the cycles, gently release the Lotus Mudra, allowing your hands to rest comfortably. Relax and breathe normally, feeling a sense of openness in your heart and throat areas, akin to the blooming of a lotus.

Upward Hand Stretch Pose Chair

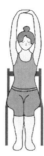

The Upward Hand Stretch Pose Chair offers a rejuvenating stretch for the upper body, making it suitable for just about anyone, anywhere. Engaging in this stretch can awaken the muscles in the shoulders and back, countering the restrictions our daily routines may place on shoulder mobility. As this movement is often neglected in daily activities, the pose helps maintain shoulder flexibility, easing tightness in the neck, back, and upper torso.

More than just a physical stretch, the pose also promotes mental relaxation and a connection to one's breath, making it an ideal warm-up before more intensive yoga sequences like the Sun Salutation Variation. Particularly valuable for older adults, this upward extension of the arms acts as a gentle heart opener, dispelling fatigue and rejuvenating the mind.

Regular practice of the Upward Hand Stretch Pose Chair can benefit those recovering from shoulder or spine injuries as part of a therapeutic regimen. It's also beneficial for those who may experience stiffness from prolonged computer use or who wish to improve posture. The uplifted arms promote better blood circulation and stimulate organs, enhancing digestive system functionality and stimulating lymph nodes in the armpits.

However, as with any yoga pose, there are precautions to consider. It may not be suitable for individuals with neck, wrists, elbows, or shoulder injuries, especially rotator cuff issues. Those with chronic pain, stiffness, or conditions like frozen shoulder should exercise caution.

Moreover, anyone recovering from surgery, even if unrelated to the upper body, should avoid this pose to prevent unintentional overstretching and potential complications.

Steps (3 minutes)

1. Begin by sitting firmly on a chair, ensuring your sit bones are anchored, and your feet are flat on the floor. Keep your back straight, and take a moment to connect with your breath.
2. Place your feet parallel to each other, spaced a few inches apart, ensuring your knees also have some distance between them. Remain in this position for 1 minute, taking grounding breaths.
3. Extend your arms in front of you and interlock your fingers, except for the index fingers, which should be extended and touching each other, forming the Kali Mudra (see p. 34).
4. Inhale, lifting your arms with the Kali Mudra above your head so they align with the crown. Exhale fully.
5. During your next inhale, slightly move your shoulders back and away from your ears, deepening the stretch in the upper back while maintaining the Kali Mudra.
6. Ensure your palms face upwards, and your hands and head are in line. Maintain your gaze forward.
7. Breathe deeply, connecting with various body parts like the chest, rib cage, upper back, and neck. Stay in this position for 1 minute and a half, stretching upward with each inhalation.
8. To release the pose, exhale and gradually lower your arms back in front of you, keeping the Kali Mudra. From this position, inhale and lift your arms again, repeating the stretch for another 1 minute and a half.
9. Conclude by returning to the initial seated position.

Seated With Eagle Arms on Chair

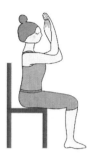

The Seated with Eagle Arms on Chair pose is a gentle Chair Yoga position, perfect especially for beginners, offering a comfortable stretch to the arms, shoulders, back, and neck. As a warm-up, this pose readies individuals for more engaging Chair Yoga sequences and can be particularly useful for strengthening the back, shoulders, and arms. Elders find this pose exceptionally advantageous, using it as a remedial practice for upper back and neck discomfort, and to keep joints in the elbows, wrists, and fingers agile, especially when facing symptoms of arthritis.

Anatomically, the pose targets and benefits muscles like the arms and shoulders, including the biceps and triceps. Though it appears simple, its benefits are manifold.

The pose stretches and strengthens the entire back, engaging the psoas and some hip muscles, as well as the core. It helps build strong shoulders and back over time.

It's a versatile pose, suitable for any location or moment. Its simplicity makes it a go-to for quick relief from shoulder or neck tension.

The pose enhances chest expansion, benefiting breathing muscles and lungs.

It improves joint flexibility, boosts blood circulation, and tones the upper arms.

Therapeutically, it aids those recovering from upper body injuries and helps alleviate symptoms of conditions like fibromyalgia and carpal tunnel syndrome.

However, there are certain cautions to be noted. Those with injuries to the neck, shoulder, or arms should practice with care or avoid it altogether. The pose might be challenging for those with cardiovascular or respiratory issues, and individuals with severe shoulder conditions like frozen shoulder should approach it with caution. The choice of chair is crucial for safety, and while it's a general practice, elders should always consult a yoga expert before diving in.

Steps (2 minutes)

1. Begin by sitting comfortably on a chair.
2. Cross your elbows, positioning the right over the left.
3. Maintain this pose for 2 minutes. As you do this, gently form the Tattva Mudra (see p. 35), with your hands by touching the tips of your index fingers to your thumbs, creating a circle, while keeping the other fingers extended. This mudra is known to encourage truthfulness and clarity in communication.

Embrace the Present Moment With Gratitude

Routine 2: Exercises for Enhanced Posture

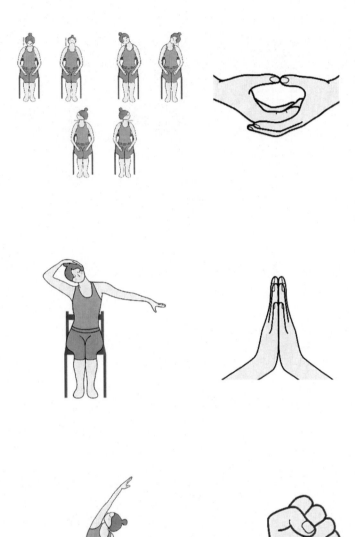

Neck Rolls Chair A-B-C with Dhyana Mudra
(3 minutes)

Begin with Neck Roll A: lower your chin to your chest and then gently tilt your head back, repeating these forward and backward movements for 1 minute. For Neck Roll B, move your head side to side, bringing your ear towards each shoulder without raising the shoulders, alternating sides for 30 seconds each. Finish with Neck Roll C: turn your head to look over each shoulder, keeping your shoulders relaxed and facing forward, again for 30 seconds each side.

Neck Stretch Chair with Apana Mudra
(2 minutes)

Sitting comfortably on a chair, close your eyes and take deep breaths to center yourself. As you inhale, raise your right arm, and lean your torso and neck gently to the left, stretching the right side. Hold this position for 1 minute, savoring the stretch. Afterward, bring your arm back down on an exhale. Repeat the movement on the other side raising your left arm and leaning to the right- Hold for 1 minute, always ensuring core engagement for stability throughout.

Seated Side Stretch Pose Chair with Mushti Mudra
(2 minutes)

Seated comfortably, close your eyes, and take a few grounding breaths. As you inhale, raise your right arm, and lean your torso to the left, stretching the right side. Hold this position, exhaling deeply and feeling the stretch. Inhale again, extending the right arm before lowering it as you exhale. Alternate between sides for 1 minute, ensuring balance and core engagement.

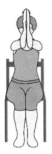 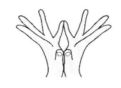

Seated Cactus Arms Together Chair with Lotus Mudra
(3 minutes)

From a seated position, inhale and raise your arms, bending at the elbows. As you exhale, press your forearms and palms together, spreading your fingers wide. Hold this position for 3 minutes.

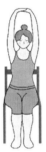 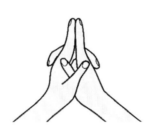

Upward Hand Stretch Pose Chair with Kali Mudra
(3 minutes)

Seated comfortably on a chair with feet grounded and spaced apart, one begins by aligning their posture and connecting to their breath. Arms are then extended and fingers interlocked, stretching them both forward and then overhead, ensuring they are in line with the head's crown. Breathing deeply, one aligns their shoulders, palms, and gaze, feeling a connection through their chest and upper back. Hold this position for 3 minutes, continuing to breathe deeply and maintain alignment.

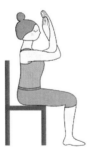 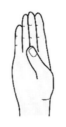

Seated with Eagle Arms on Chair with Tattva Mudra
(2 minutes)

Seated on a chair, intertwine your arms with the right side dominant. Hold the position for 1 minute. Then, switch to have the left side dominant and maintain the position for another 1 minute, emphasizing coordination and awareness throughout the practice.

Enhancing Leg Strength and Mobility

Our legs play a crucial role in the journey to maintain physical well-being, especially as we age. They don't just support the weight of our body but also facilitate movement, making it essential to ensure they stay strong and agile. This chapter delves deep into the importance of leg strength and mobility, particularly in the context of older adults who are more prone to issues like muscle atrophy, reduced joint flexibility, and balance challenges.

Chair Yoga emerges as a beacon of hope in this scenario. It offers a series of poses specifically focusing on the legs, targeting muscles from the thighs to the calves and even the intricate muscles around the hips. These poses strengthen the muscles and enhance flexibility, ensuring a broader and more comfortable range of motion. Moreover, with consistent practice, these exercises can help improve circulation, reduce the risk of leg cramps, and even mitigate the onset of conditions like osteoporosis.

However, it's not solely a matter of strength and flexibility. A significant part of leg health revolves around balance. As we delve further into this chapter, you'll discover poses that focus on equilibrium, an essential aspect of preventing falls, a common concern among older adults.

Finally, we address some common leg and hip concerns often encountered by older individuals. From the discomfort of arthritis to the challenges of limited mobility, Chair Yoga offers solutions that are not only effective but also accessible, ensuring that age is never a barrier to a healthier, more mobile life.

Join us in this chapter as we explore the transformative power of Chair Yoga for leg strength and mobility, offering a renewed sense of independence and vitality.

Routine for Preventing Falls and Improving Balance

Balance is pivotal in preventing falls, a concern often magnified in older adults due to weakening muscles and reduced reflexes. This routine incorporates a series of poses aimed at enhancing leg strength, stability, and proprioception. By regularly engaging with these poses, practitioners can expect to see improvements in their balance, instilling confidence in movement and reducing the risk of falls.

Targeted Exercises for Leg and Hip Wellness

The legs and hips can be areas of discomfort, particularly with the onset of conditions like arthritis or due to sedentary lifestyles. This routine delves into poses tailored to stretch, strengthen, and alleviate discomfort in the hip and leg region. The poses also promote better circulation, flexibility, and joint health. Adopting this routine can mitigate common leg and hip concerns, facilitate pain-free movement, and improve joint function.

Each routine is designed to be 15 minutes long, featuring six poses. However, it is important to listen to your body. If you find it challenging to maintain a pose for the indicated time, do not worry. Hold each pose for as long as you feel comfortable, and with practice, you will gradually increase your endurance. There is no rush and no pressure—your comfort and safety are the most important.

Routine 1: Preventing Falls and Improving Balance

Flexing Foot Pose Chair

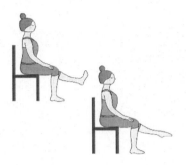

The Flexing Foot Pose is a seated exercise focusing on foot and ankle joint movements. While seated on a chair, participants engage in two primary foot movements: dorsiflexion, drawing the foot closer to the leg, stretching the calf muscles, and plantar flexion, where the foot moves downward like pressing a car's gas pedal. This pose is particularly favored as a warm-up, especially by athletes and runners, to nurture foot health. It's also a soothing cooldown for tired legs.

This pose proves especially useful in Chair Yoga sequences, offering a practical option for those who might find standing on one leg or sitting on the floor challenging. It's ideal for individuals with ligament issues in the knees and ankles, those recovering from Achilles tendonitis, or those recuperating from leg surgeries or injuries. Interestingly, this variation can also be performed while lying in bed, ensuring muscle mobility for those confined for extended periods due to illness. Its gentle nature helps prevent muscle cramps and stiffness, making it a valuable addition to desk yoga, prenatal routines, or daily stretches in preparation for an active day.

Anatomically, this pose primarily benefits the feet, ankles, hamstrings, and quadriceps. Regarding its benefits, the Flexing Foot Pose Chair serves as an alternative to typical warm-ups, with the chair providing essential support. This pose is particularly helpful for those prone to dizziness when executing similar movements while standing. It's suitable for older adults and even those confined to bed due to illness. Additionally, individuals undergoing rehabilitation post-accident, injury, surgery, or those with conditions like Achilles tendonitis or plantar fasciitis can benefit from this pose. The gentle movements aid in strengthening the involved joints and muscles, promoting healthy blood flow. This pose can also be conveniently practiced at a desk, during travel stops, or before intense physical activities.

However, there are some considerations. While generally safe for all, those recovering from foot or ankle strains, sprains, and fractures should proceed with caution. Individuals with foot and ankle arthritis, older adults, or those recuperating from injuries should avoid rapid movements. Those experiencing back pain might consider supporting their back with a rolled blanket for added comfort. Lastly, ensuring a sturdy chair is crucial, and additional props like pillows or bolsters might be useful for foot support.

Steps (2 minutes)

1. Start by taking a seat on a chair. Extend your spine, close your eyes, and relax. Place your hands on your thighs with the palms facing up, ready to form the Apana Mudra (see p. 41).
2. To create the Apana Mudra, join the tips of your thumbs, middle fingers, and ring fingers on each hand, leaving the other fingers extended. This mudra is known for aiding in the elimination process and regulating the downward flow of energy.
3. As you inhale, gently lift your left leg to an angle of about 40 degrees, ensuring your right foot remains grounded on the floor. Keep your hands in the Apana Mudra on your thighs.
4. While maintaining the lifted position of your left leg, inhale and flex the ankle and toes of your left foot up and down. Continue this flexing motion for 1 minute, synchronizing it with your breath.
5. After completing the repetitions, keep your left foot elevated in the air for a few breaths, feeling a stretch in the Achilles tendon. Maintain the Apana Mudra,

focusing on the flow of energy and relaxation.

6. Gently lower the left leg back to the floor, still keeping your hands in the Apana Mudra.
7. Repeat the same flexing process with your right leg, lifting it and flexing the ankle and toes for 1 minute.
8. Ensure careful movement when flexing the ankle and toes, especially if there's existing inflammation. If the movement causes discomfort, avoid it entirely, focusing instead on maintaining the Apana Mudra and relaxed breathing.

Seated Half Wind Release Pose I Chair

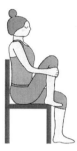

The Seated Half Wind Release Pose is a gentle chair yoga posture that offers a variety of health benefits, particularly targeting the knees, pelvic area, and the psoas muscle—crucial components for maintaining lower body mobility and core strength.

As you settle into the Seated Half Wind Release Pose, you gently draw one knee towards the chest, which can help in releasing tension in the lower back and pelvic region. The action of holding the knee close to the body engages the psoas muscle, which is vital for hip flexibility and stability. Regular practice of this pose can lead to enhanced joint health and can be a soothing balm for those experiencing digestive discomfort, as it stimulates abdominal organs.

The Seated Half Wind Release Pose is a staple in chair yoga sequences, where the support of the chair allows practitioners of all levels to enjoy the stretch without strain. It's also a common feature in restorative yoga classes, where the focus is on relaxing the body and calming the mind.

While the Seated Half Wind Release Pose is generally considered safe and beneficial, it's important to know your body's signals. If you have any knee or hip concerns, you should approach this pose with caution. It's always best to consult with a healthcare professional or a certified yoga instructor before incorporating new poses into your practice, particularly if you have any existing health issues or concerns.

Steps (2 minutes)

1. Sit upright on a chair, grounding your feet firmly.
2. Place your hands on your knees or the armrests for support.
3. Smoothly draw your right knee toward your chest.
4. Encircle your shin or back of the thigh with your hands, whichever feels more comfortable.
5. Gently hold your right knee, inviting a soft stretch into the lower back and hip area.
6. As you hold the pose, form the Tattva Mudra (see p. 35), by bringing the tip of your thumb and index finger together, creating a circle, while extending the other fingers straight out. Do this with both hands, whether they are on the shin or thigh.
7. Breathe deeply, allowing the abdomen to press against the thigh on each inhale, enhancing the stretch.
8. Maintain this gentle embrace for 1 minute, tuning into the body's subtle release with each exhale.
9. Carefully lower your right leg, return to the starting position, and feel the release in your hip and lower back.
10. Switch to the left leg, repeating the mindful movements and mudra, holding the stretch for 1 minute to foster balance in the practice.
11. Conclude with both feet flat on the ground, hands resting with the Tattva Mudra, taking a moment to breathe and integrate the stretch's effects.

Wide-Legged Seated Twist Chair

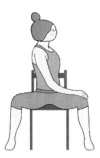

The Wide-Legged Seated Twist Chair offers a gentle yet effective twist that is ideal for yoga beginners or those with limited mobility. Performed while sitting on a chair with legs spread wide, this approach uniquely achieves flexibility and relief and is specifically designed for Chair Yoga sequences. It's particularly beneficial for older adults or those engaged in restorative and prenatal yoga.

This pose focuses not only on twisting to open the heart but also allows hip opening, providing dual benefits for both the upper and lower body. As a warmup, it's effective in elongating the spine and expanding chest muscles, providing significant relief for those often seated or involved in sports. It's especially useful for people with poor posture, as it eases back pain and stiffness in the neck and shoulders. Practiced daily, it can also enhance detoxification processes, potentially boosting immunity.

Anatomically, this pose targets the upper limbs, shoulders, and the entire back, from the lower to the upper region. It also works on the chest and hips, especially the external hip region, and even the knees.

Although the pose is widespread in Chair Yoga, prenatal yoga, restorative yoga, and sequences focused on heart and hip opening, its benefits are manifold. The grounding effect of wide legs combined with the twist offers a gentle stretch around the knees, lower back, and pelvic floor, strengthening them in the process. The chair's support allows for a deeper twist, enhancing flexibility in the waist and lower body. This pose not only lengthens the spine but also activates the chest, rib, upper back, and shoulder muscles, promoting deeper breathing and serving as a gentle heart opener. Engaging the pelvis and psoas muscles, this pose helps maintain proper posture, alleviating tightness in the neck, back, hips, and legs.

However, despite its many advantages, there are precautions to consider. It's crucial to be cautious if one has had any surgeries or injuries related to the abdomen, pelvic floor, lower back, or any part of the upper body, including the neck, shoulders, and ribcage. Those with high or low blood pressure, heart ailments, or severe conditions like Inflammatory Bowel Disease should also exercise caution. Students with stiffness in the neck or shoulders should warm up appropriately. Lastly, the choice of chair is crucial; one without arms is preferable to facilitate the pose effectively.

Steps (3 minutes)

1. Sit on a chair, extending your spine and closing your eyes to relax. Let your hands rest on your thighs in a relaxed position.
2. Sit with your spine erect and spread your legs wide apart for comfort and balance.
3. Take a deep breath in. As you do so, form the Mushti Mudra (see p. 39), by clenching your fists, and keeping your thumbs inside the fingers. This mudra is known for releasing pent-up emotions and tension.
4. As you exhale, gently twist your upper body to the right, using your left hand on the right knee to aid the twist. Feel the release of tension as you maintain the mudra.
5. Hold this position for 1 minute and a half, feeling the stretch across the spine and hips, and experiencing the emotional release facilitated by the Mushti Mudra.
6. Inhale as you return to the center position, releasing the Mushti Mudra

momentarily.

7. Exhale and prepare to repeat the twist on the left side. Form the Mushti Mudra again with your right hand and use it on the left knee for support as you twist.

8. Hold this position and breathe deeply for 1 minute and a half, feeling the stretch and the emotional cleansing effect of the Mushti Mudra.

9. Return to the center and relax, unclenching your fists and allowing the benefits of the pose and mudra to sink in. Breathe deeply and feel a sense of relaxation and emotional release.

Seated External Hip Rotation Pose Chair

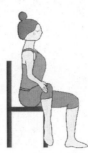

The Seated External Hip Rotation Pose Chair primarily focuses on benefiting the muscles around the hips and knees. This pose targets the external hip rotators, enhancing flexibility and mobility in these often tense areas. Practicing this pose can help alleviate tension and stiffness accumulated from daily activities or prolonged sitting.

It is particularly beneficial for those who may find traditional floor-based poses challenging.

Beyond its physical benefits, this pose can also help prepare the body for deeper hip-opening poses, making it a valuable addition to hip-focused sequences.

However, while the Seated External Hip Rotation Pose Chair offers numerous advantages, it is crucial to practice with caution. Individuals with existing hip or knee issues should approach this pose carefully, and it is always recommended to consult with a yoga instructor or therapist to ensure the practice is safe and beneficial.

Steps (2 minutes)

1. Locate a chair where you can sit comfortably with your spine in an upright position and your feet resting flat on the ground.
2. Ensure that your knees are in line with your ankles, creating a 90-degree angle.
3. Take a deep breath in, getting ready for the motion.
4. While exhaling, softly raise your right foot off the floor.
5. Position your right ankle over your left knee, forming a figure-four shape with your legs.
6. Maintain a flexed position with your right foot to safeguard the knee joint.
7. As your hands rest, create the Jala Mudra (see p. 42), by gently bringing together the tips of your thumb and little finger while keeping the other three fingers extended. This mudra is recognized for its ability to harmonize the water elements within the body. Depending on your comfort, you can place your hands with the Jala Mudra on your lap or the chair's armrests.
8. Maintain an upright posture, sensing the stretch in your right hip.
9. Take deep breaths and sustain this position for 1 minute.
10. Softly return your right foot to the floor.
11. Repeat the procedure using your left leg, holding the position for 1 minute.
12. After performing the exercise on both sides, return to a neutral seated position and pause to observe the sensations in your hips and legs.

Staff Pose Chair II

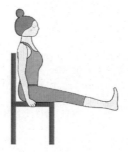

Staff Pose Chair II is a seated posture that offers an accessible way to experience the benefits of the traditional Staff Pose, especially suitable for those who find floor exercises challenging. By practicing this pose in a chair, individuals can more effectively target key muscle groups.

In Staff Pose Chair II, the primary muscles that are activated and stretched include the hamstrings, hips, and quadriceps. It makes the pose particularly beneficial for anyone looking to improve the flexibility and strength of these muscle groups.

Due to its seated nature, it's a popular choice in Chair Yoga routines, making yoga accessible to people with mobility limitations. Additionally, its gentle stretching of the hips and hamstrings makes it a valuable addition to prenatal and postnatal yoga sessions. Furthermore, the pose can be used in hip-opening sequences, allowing for gradual and controlled stretching of the hip muscles.

While the specific benefits of Staff Pose Chair II are not listed, based on its muscle focus, one can infer that it aids in lengthening and strengthening the hamstrings, hips, and quadriceps. It could improve posture, alleviate discomfort in the lower back, and prepare the body for more advanced poses. Additionally, the seated nature of this pose on a chair allows for greater stability and support, making it accessible to a wider range of practitioners.

Detailed contraindications for Staff Pose Chair II are not provided here. However, as with any yoga pose, individuals should approach it cautiously if they have any existing injuries, especially in the hips, hamstrings, or quadriceps. It's advisable to seek guidance from a healthcare professional or an experienced yoga instructor before trying out new poses, particularly if you have any health concerns.

Steps (3 minutes)

1. As you sit in the pose with your spine extended and feet grounded, bring your hands up to chest level.
2. In the Vitarka Mudra (see p. 37), form a circle with the thumb and index finger of each hand, keeping the other fingers extended. This mudra is often associated with the transmission of Buddha's teachings and is said to symbolize intellectual discussion or argument.
3. With your palms facing outward, rest the hands in front of your chest, maintaining the mudra. Ensure your shoulders remain relaxed and your spine stays elongated.
4. As you hold the Staff Pose with the Vitarka Mudra, focus on the flow of your breath and the sense of openness and clarity this gesture symbolizes.
5. Continue to breathe deeply, maintaining the pose and the mudra for 3 minutes.
6. Upon completion, gently lower your hands back to your sides or the chair's armrests and release the mudra, returning to a neutral seated position.

Seated Windshield Wiper Pose Chair

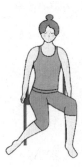

The Seated Windshield Wiper Pose, when practiced in a chair, is a gentle movement that offers a variety of anatomical benefits. It primarily focuses on the hips, the inner hip area, knees, and the psoas muscle, promoting flexibility and strength in these areas.

From a categorization standpoint, this pose is primarily seen as a warm-up exercise, preparing the body for more intense postures or sequences. Furthermore, given its hip-opening nature, it's also incorporated into prenatal yoga sequences, offering relief and flexibility to expectant mothers.

The benefits of the Seated Windshield Wiper Pose Chair are manifold. While the specific advantages aren't detailed here, it's reasonable to infer from its targeted muscles that the pose aids in releasing tension from the hips, enhancing joint mobility, and stretching the psoas muscle. It can be particularly helpful for those who spend long hours seated, as it alleviates stiffness and promotes better posture.

However, like all yoga poses, the Seated Windshield Wiper Pose Chair comes with certain contraindications. It's essential to be aware of any physical limitations or conditions that might make this pose inadvisable. Always consult with a qualified yoga instructor or healthcare professional if unsure.

Steps (3 minutes)

1. Start by sitting comfortably on a chair, ensuring your feet are firmly planted on the floor. Maintain an upright spine and relaxed shoulders.
2. Create the Vayu Mudra (see p. 36): Gently fold the index finger of each hand towards the palm and press it with the thumb, while leaving the other fingers extended. This mudra is thought to harmonize the air element within the body, fostering both physical and mental relaxation.
3. Place your hands with the Vayu Mudra on your knees or the edges of the chair for stability.
4. Gently move both knees to the right side, simulating the movement of windshield wipers. Keep your movements slow and controlled, focusing on the sensation in your hips.
5. Return your knees to the center position.
6. Repeat the movement, this time moving both knees to the left side. Feel the gentle stretch and rotation in your lower back and hips.
7. Return to the center position once more, maintaining the Vayu Mudra and your upright posture.
8. Continue to move your knees from side to side, maintaining a rhythmic motion. Remember to breathe deeply and evenly throughout the exercise.
9. Ensure your feet remain flat on the ground throughout the movement, providing stability and grounding.
10. After 3 minutes, come back to a neutral seated position and relax. Take a moment to notice any changes in your body, particularly around the hips and lower back where you've been working. Release the Vayu Mudra gently.

Routine 1: Preventing Falls and Improving Balance

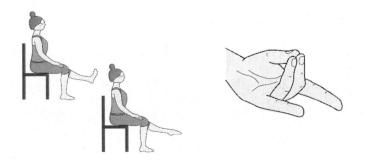

Flexing Foot Pose Chair with Apana Mudra
(2 minutes)

Seated on a chair, transition from a relaxed state to lifting one leg at a 40-degree angle. Flex the ankle and toes of the elevated leg up and down, repeating this about 1 minute. Feel the stretch in the Achilles tendon before switching to the other leg. Practice with caution, especially if inflammation is present.

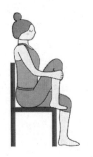
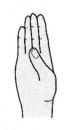

Seated Half Wind Release Pose I Chair with Tattva Mudra
(2 minutes)

Sit with a poised posture on the edge of your chair, feet pressing into the earth. Extend your arms forward, shoulder level, and gracefully hinge at the hips, folding forward with the elegance of a willow. Rest your forearms on your thighs for a gentle anchor, heels lifted in playful preparation as if tiptoeing on air. Breathe into this shape, feeling the stretch whisper through your back and legs, a silent symphony of movement and stillness. Hold this position for 1 minute on each side, alternating between the right and left sides. When you're ready to return, do so easily, rolling up to sit tall, feet returning to their grounded dance with the floor.

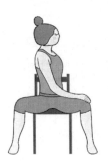
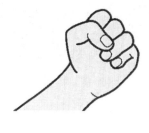

Wide-Legged Seated Twist Chair with Mushti Mudra
(3 minutes)

Take a deep inhalation, seated on a chair with legs spread wide for balance. As you exhale, gently rotate your torso to the right, guiding the twist with your left hand on the right knee. After savoring the stretch across your spine and hips for 1 minute and a half, return to center on an inhalation. Repeat the twist towards the left, using your right hand for guidance. Conclude by settling back into a centered, relaxed position, letting the invigorating effects of the twist permeate your body.

All pose images are copyright by Tummee - sequencing platform for yoga teachers

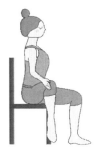 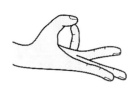

Seated External Hip Rotation Pose Chair with Jala Mudra
(2 minutes)

Seated on a comfortable chair with a straight spine and feet grounded. Lift one foot and place its ankle over the opposite knee in a figure four configuration. With the lifted foot flexed to ensure knee safety, the practitioner sits tall, feeling a gentle stretch in the hip. Hands rest gracefully on the lap or chair's armrests. Deep breaths enhance the stretch, providing relaxation. After 1 minute, the pose is repeated with the other leg, offering balanced flexibility.

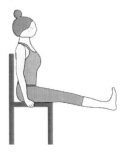 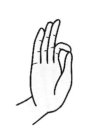

Staff Pose Chair II with Vitarka Mudra
(3 minutes)

Sitting firmly on a chair with feet grounded, align your knees above your ankles. With a tall spine stretching from base to crown, place your hands by your hips and engage your core. Shoulders remain relaxed, neck in alignment with the spine. As you press down through the sit bones, elongate the spine further. Holding this posture for 3 minutes, breathe deeply, emphasizing a lengthened stature. After soaking in the pose, ease back into a relaxed seated position.

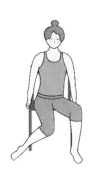 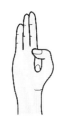

Seated Windshield Wiper Pose Chair with Vayu Mudra
(3 minutes)

Sit upright on a chair and rhythmically move the knees from side to side, akin to the swiping of windshield wipers. The repetitive motion aids in hip mobility, especially beneficial for those with sedentary lifestyles. Continue this motion for 3 minutes. By the end of the sequence, one finds relaxation and a subtle release in the hip region.

All pose images are copyright by Tummee - sequencing platform for yoga teachers

Routine 2: Targeted Exercises for Leg and Hip Wellness

Half Seated Forward Bend Pose Chair

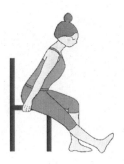

The Half-Seated Forward Bend Pose Chair is a yoga posture offering various benefits for different muscle groups and is often incorporated into specific yoga sequences. This pose engages various muscle groups in a gentle and seated position.

During the Half-Seated Forward Bend Pose Chair, you engage your arm muscles, including the biceps and triceps, as you stretch forward and extend your arms. This action helps strengthen your upper arms.

Your feet and ankle muscles are also involved in maintaining stability and support while performing this pose. They aid in grounding your body, providing a sense of balance and foundation.

This pose provides a gentle stretch to the hamstrings and the muscles at the back of your thighs. Regular practice can help improve flexibility in that area, making it easier to carry out various physical activities.

The muscles of the front thigh, known as the quadriceps, are also engaged as they work to maintain the position of your legs during the pose. This engagement helps build strength in the quadriceps.

The Half-Seated Forward Bend Pose Chair is commonly included in Chair Yoga sequences. This variation of yoga is particularly suitable for individuals who may have mobility issues or prefer practicing yoga in a seated position using a chair for support.

Regarding benefits, regular practice of the Half Seated Forward Bend Pose Chair can lead to improved flexibility, especially in the hamstrings and lower back. It strengthens the arm muscles, particularly the biceps and triceps. Additionally, it encourages proper alignment and posture by stretching and elongating the spine. Like many yoga poses, it promotes relaxation and stress relief, helping calm the mind.

However, it's important to note that this pose might not be suitable for everyone. Individuals with severe back issues or recent surgeries should exercise caution or consult with a healthcare professional or experienced yoga instructor. Similarly, those with knee problems or severe balance issues may need to modify the pose or seek guidance to ensure their safety during practice. Always prioritize safety and listen to your body when practicing yoga.

Steps (2 minutes)

1. Sit comfortably on a chair, ensuring that your spine is erect and your feet are flat on the ground.
2. Move your thighs forward and gently extend your right leg, placing the right foot on the floor with the heel resting on the ground.
3. Point your toes upward, pressing your heel firmly into the ground. This action stretches the sole of your foot. Feel the stretch along the inner sole and maintain this position for about 6 breaths.
4. While in this position, focus on extending and stretching the quadriceps, hamstrings, and calves, along with the soles of your feet.
5. While maintaining the stretch, form the Mushti Mudra (see p. 39), by clenching your fists. This mudra helps channel energy and release pent-up emotions or stress. Hold this mudra gently, without straining your hands.

6. After holding the position and mudra for 1 minute, gently release the stretch, unclench your fists, and relax.
7. Now repeat the same sequence with your left leg. Hold the position longer to maximize the stretch and benefits if one of your legs has more issues or tension.
8. After completing the stretches on both sides, gently release the stretch and return to a neutral seated position. Allow both feet to rest flat on the floor and pause briefly to become aware of the sensations.

Ankle Crank on Chair

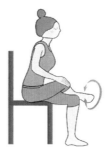

The Ankle Crank On Chair pose is a yoga warm-up designed to ready the body for more intense yoga poses and flows. This pose mainly benefits the muscles in the feet and ankles, making it a fitting choice for sequences that focus on these muscle groups. It also involves the hips.

Classified as a warm-up, it's the ideal option for sequences that aim to enhance the body's flexibility and mobility gradually.

While specific benefits and contraindications for the Ankle Crank On Chair pose aren't listed here, they're crucial to consider when incorporating this pose into your practice. Understanding the benefits underscores its contribution to overall wellbeing, while being aware of contraindications ensures safe practice, avoiding potential issues.

Adding the Ankle Crank On Chair pose to your yoga routine can be extremely valuable, particularly for warming up and targeting the feet, ankles, and hips.

Steps (2 minutes)

1. Begin by sitting in the Dandasana position on a chair, ensuring you are comfortable and your spine is straight.
2. Rest your right foot on your left knee, allowing it to dangle freely.
3. As you prepare to rotate your ankle, form the Vitarka Mudra (see p. 37) with your hands. To do this, touch the tips of your thumb and index finger together, forming a circle while keeping the other fingers extended. This mudra is often associated with the transmission of spiritual knowledge and is believed to improve focus.
4. Inhale deeply and begin rotating your right ankle. Start with clockwise movements for 1 minute.
5. Keeping the Vitarka Mudra intact, continue to breathe evenly and maintain a straight back to ensure proper posture.
6. After completing clockwise rotations, proceed with anticlockwise rotations for another 1 minute.
7. Gently release your right foot down and switch to the left foot, resting it on your right knee. Repeat the ankle rotations while maintaining the Vitarka Mudra.
8. As you rotate your ankles, focus on the sensation in your calves, inner soles, and sides of your lower legs. The Vitarka Mudra can help center your attention, enhancing the meditative aspect of the movement.
9. This combination of ankle movement and hand gesture can foster a sense of tranquility and concentration, while also promoting physical benefits such as smoother and more flexible ankle joints. It can be particularly beneficial for those with arthritis, aiding in reducing pain and swelling.
10. Conclude the exercise by bringing both feet back to the ground, and releasing the mudra, taking a moment to observe the effects of the practice on your body and mind.

Goddess Pose with Arms Down

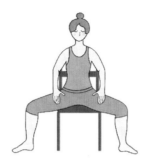

The Goddess Pose with Arms Down involves using a chair as a prop. This adaptation offers several benefits and is suitable for a range of practitioners, including beginners and those with specific needs.

In this pose, practitioners stand beside a chair with their feet positioned wide apart, mirroring the wide-legged stance of the traditional Goddess Pose. The chair provides support and stability, making it accessible for those who may have limitations in strength, flexibility, or balance.

The Goddess Pose with Arms Down, aided by a chair, provides a gentle hip opener that relieves tension in the lower body and back, making it ideal for beginners and those with mobility challenges. It enhances mindfulness, improves alignment, and strengthens the legs, core, and back. This pose is excellent for therapeutic yoga, particularly beneficial for seniors and individuals with stiff hips and backs. It's a valuable addition to desk yoga routines, helping to ease stiffness from prolonged sitting. Additionally, its adaptability makes it suitable for people with special needs, offering a safe and accessible yoga option.

The Goddess Pose with Arms Down is a beneficial yoga variation, yet certain precautions are essential. It's not recommended for individuals with recent injuries or surgeries involving the hamstrings, ankles, feet, or hips. Those with weaker bone structures, joint issues, or conditions like fibromyalgia should approach this pose with caution, especially if experiencing discomfort in the lower back, hips, or legs. It's important to consult with a yoga instructor before attempting the pose. Additionally, choosing the right chair, preferably one with a back and without armrests, is crucial for safety and comfort. While this pose offers various benefits, individuals with specific health concerns should always seek professional advice to ensure safe practice.

Steps (3 minutes)

1. Begin by sitting in a wide-legged position on a chair.
2. Place your feet wide apart.
3. Engage your core and maintain an upright posture.
4. Form the Jala Mudra (see p. 42), by touching the tips of your thumb and little finger together on both hands, while extending the other three fingers.
5. With the Jala Mudra formed, hold your hands either in front of your lower abdomen or let them rest comfortably by your sides, depending on what feels more balanced.
6. As you hold the pose, focus on feeling the stretch in your hips and lower body, integrating the calming energy of the Jala Mudra, which is believed to balance the water element in the body.
7. Breathe deeply and steadily, maintaining the position and the mudra for 3 minutes. Concentrate on the sensation of fluidity and ease that the Jala Mudra may introduce to your practice.

Knee Head Down Chair

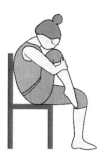

The Knee Head Down Chair is a yoga posture offering a range of benefits, primarily focusing on specific muscle groups. This pose is commonly integrated into various types of yoga sequences, including Chair Yoga, restorative yoga, and hip-opening yoga. The Knee Head Down Chair pose offers a comprehensive workout, particularly benefiting the lower body. It effectively engages and strengthens the gluteal muscles, which are essential for hip stability and mobility. By enhancing the strength of these muscles, the pose contributes to overall lower body strength.

Additionally, the pose is effective in promoting increased mobility in the hips, encouraging a broader range of motion that can be especially beneficial for individuals aiming to improve their flexibility and reduce stiffness in the hip area. For those with knee concerns or injuries, this pose is particularly valuable as it supports the knees, thereby reducing strain on the knee joints and aiding in overall knee health.

Although specific contraindications for the Knee Head Down Chair aren't provided here, exercising caution when attempting this pose is crucial, especially if you have existing hip, knee, or back issues. It is advisable to seek guidance from a certified yoga instructor or a healthcare professional to determine whether the pose is appropriate and safe for your circumstances and requirements.

Steps (2 minutes)

1. Begin sitting comfortably with a straight spine.
2. Gently lift your right leg off the chair, drawing your right thigh close to your chest. If necessary, use your hands or yoga straps for support to bring the thigh closer, especially if flexibility or body weight makes this challenging.
3. As you hold your right thigh close, let's integrate the Tattva Mudra (see p. 35). To do this movement, bring your hands together in front of your chest in a prayer position. Connect the tips of your thumbs and index fingers, forming a circle, while the other fingers remain extended. This mudra symbolizes truth and honesty and can help foster a sense of inner integrity and clarity during your practice.
4. While maintaining the Tattva Mudra, focus on the movement of knee flexion and hip engagement. This helps in keeping the joints active and healthy. The pose, combined with the mudra, can also aid in a quicker recovery after a fall or injury to the hip or knee, as well as promote a deeper sense of truthfulness in your practice.
5. Keep your breathing steady and deep, focusing on the stretch's sensation and the mudra's symbolism.
6. After holding the pose for 1 minute, gently release your right leg back to the floor and release the mudra.
7. Repeat the same sequence with your left leg, ensuring to maintain the Tattva Mudra during the pose.

Easy Pose Chair One Leg Raised

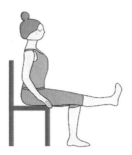

The Easy Pose Chair One Leg Raised involves sitting on a chair while maintaining an upright back and feet flat on the ground. You then enter the Easy Pose by crossing one leg over the other, placing your feet beneath your knees. Lift one leg off the ground while keeping the other foot firmly anchored on the chair, engaging the muscles of the raised foot and ankle for balance.

The Easy Pose Chair One Leg Raised in Chair Yoga is a gentle yet effective exercise for enhancing foot and ankle strength, improving balance, and increasing flexibility in the hips and knees. Ideal for Chair Yoga, it's particularly beneficial for individuals with limited mobility or those who find standing yoga poses challenging.

However, caution is advised for those with severe ankle or knee injuries, as this pose may aggravate their condition. If discomfort, pain, or dizziness occurs during the practice, it's important to stop and consult a healthcare professional or yoga instructor. Practicing this pose mindfully and within your body's limits is crucial to ensure safety and avoid any discomfort.

Steps (3 minutes)

1. Begin by sitting on a chair, positioning half of your thighs on the chair while keeping your back away from the backrest. Ensure your spine is upright for proper posture.
2. Sit up straight, focusing on relaxed breathing. Place your feet firmly on the floor, ensuring your entire feet are grounded, not just the toes.
3. As you inhale, gently lift your right leg so that it is parallel to the floor. Point your toes upward, striving to keep your leg as straight as possible.
4. While maintaining this position, tighten your knees and quadriceps. Coordinate your breathing with the pose: inhale deeply and exhale slowly. Hold this position for 1 minute and a half.
5. As you hold the pose, form the Apana Mudra (see p. 41), with your hands. To perform this mudra, join the tips of your thumb, middle finger, and ring finger together while keeping the other fingers extended. This mudra is thought to assist in the elimination process and is associated with a grounding effect.
6. Maintain focus on the stretch in your ankles, soles, and calves. If you also feel the stretch in the back of your knee and hamstrings, gently shift your attention to the soles and calves, where the stretch should be more prominent.
7. After holding for 1 minute and a half, gently release your right leg, lowering it back to the floor.
8. Repeat the same sequence with your left leg, continuing to use the Apana Mudra with your hands for balance and focus.
9. Once you have completed the sequence with both legs, relax and return to a neutral seated position. Take a moment to notice any sensations in your body, especially in the areas you have been stretching.

Seated Hip Circle Chair

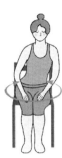

The Seated Hip Circle Chair is a chair-based yoga practice where you perform circular hip movements while seated. It's akin to Standing Pelvic Circles but adapted for the limited range of motion available when seated on a chair. This variation is commonly included in yoga sequences for older adults, offering them a way to strengthen their hips even with limited flexibility.

Gently rotating the hips in circular motions helps relieve daily tension that tends to accumulate in the hip area, particularly for those who spend long hours sitting at desks. It makes it suitable for corporate yoga sessions, addressing the impact of modern sedentary lifestyles.

This practice can boost energy levels and is suitable for inclusion in dynamic yoga sequences.

Steps (3 minutes)

1. Start by ensuring your feet are firmly grounded on the floor while seated on the chair.
2. Ensure both sit bones are firmly fixed on the seat with equal weight distribution.
3. Keep your head aligned with your spine. Position your hands on your thighs, ensuring your spine remains upright and attentive.
4. Form the Dhyana Mudra (see p. 40), with the right hand on top of the left, palms facing up, and the tips of the thumbs gently touching. This mudra symbolizes meditation and concentration.
5. Take a deep breath in, engage your core by pulling your belly button toward your spine, and elevate your ribcage to sustain proper posture.
6. Breathe gently and with awareness. If comfortable, close your eyes to enhance focus.
7. Inhale and lengthen your torso upward from the pelvis. Begin to rotate your upper body in smooth circles, guided by the hips.
8. Although the range of motion may be limited, focus on making controlled and aware movements.
9. Rotate in a smooth clockwise circular motion for 1 minute and a half, then switch to counterclockwise for another 1 minute and a half.
10. Coordinate your breath with the movement; inhale as you move forward and exhale as you move backward.
11. Maintain a slow and steady rhythm, focusing on stability and comfort in the hip movement.

Inner Peace Is a New Strength

Routine 2: Targeted Exercises for Leg and Hip Wellness

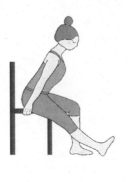 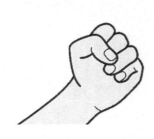

Half Seated Forward Bend Pose Chair with Mushti Mudra
(2 minutes)

This seated Chair Yoga pose stretches the soles of your feet and lower leg muscles. Extend one leg, press the heel down, and point your toes up, feeling the stretch. Hold this position for 1 minute working on quadriceps, hamstrings, and calves. Repeat with the other leg. Relax and return to a seated position.

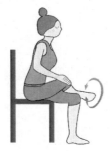 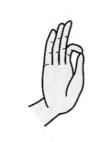

Ankle Crank on Chair with Vitarka Mudra
(2 minutes)

Sit on the chair, cross your right foot over the left knee, and let it hang freely. Rotate your ankle clockwise and anticlockwise for approximately 1 minute each. Switch to the left foot over the right knee and repeat the ankle rotations. Focus on feeling the stretch in your calves, inner soles, and the sides of your lower leg as you perform these rotations.

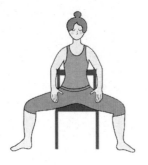 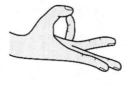

Goddess Pose with Arms Down with Jala Mudra
(3 minutes)

Begin by sitting on a chair in a wide-legged position, feet spread apart. Engage your core and sit up straight. You can either hold your hands in front of your lower abdomen or let them rest by your sides. As you maintain this pose, focus on the stretch in your hips and lower body. Breathe deeply and steadily, holding the pose for 3 minutes, and immerse yourself in the sense of fluidity and ease it brings to your practice.

All pose images are copyright by Tummee - sequencing platform for yoga teachers

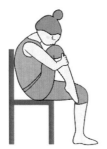 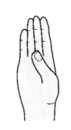

Knee Head Down Chair with Tattva Mudra
(2 minutes)

In the Knee Head Down Chair pose, begin from Pigeon Pose Chair (see p. 59). Lift your right leg off the chair, gently drawing your right thigh close to your chest. If this movement feels challenging due to body weight or flexibility, you can use your hands to support the thigh. Hold this position for 2 minutes.

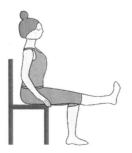 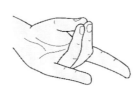

Easy Pose Chair One Leg Raised with Apana Mudra
(3 minutes)

Sit on a chair with half of your thighs on the chair and maintain an upright posture without leaning your back against the chair for support. Keep your feet firmly planted on the floor, ensuring that the entire soles of your feet are in contact with the ground. As you inhale, raise your right leg until it is parallel to the floor, with your toes pointing upward and your leg as straight as possible. Tighten your knees and quadriceps while coordinating your breath, and hold this position for 1 minute and a half. Repeat with your left leg.

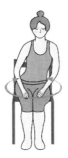 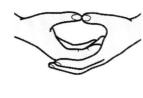

Seated Hip Circle Chair with Dhyana Mudra
(3 minutes)

Sit comfortably on a chair with feet grounded, ensuring even weight distribution on the seat. Keep your spine straight and your hands on your thighs. Inhale deeply, engage your core, and gently rotate your upper body in controlled circles from your hips, first clockwise for 1 minute and a half, then counterclockwise for another 1 minute and a half. Coordinate your breathing with the movement, maintaining a stable, focused rhythm.

Chapter 8: Chair Yoga Regimens: Tailored for Results

15-Day Chair Yoga Journey: Training and Progress Tracking

Welcome aboard your 15-day Chair Yoga adventure! This program is your guide to a variety of chair yoga routines, each crafted to boost not just your physical health but also your mental well-being. Over these next 15 days, you're not just going to enhance your flexibility and strength; you're also going to dive deep into the versatility of yoga and how it can be customized to match your unique needs and likes.

Days 1 to 5: Laying Down the Foundations

The first leg of our journey is all about building a solid base in chair yoga. We'll start with the basics: grounding techniques, simple poses, and breathing exercises. Think of these first five days as your yoga 'getting-to-know-you' phase. It's about getting comfy with the practice, nailing the alignment of each pose, and prepping your body for the more advanced stuff that's to come.

Days 6 to 10: Boosting Strength in Upper and Lower Body

Now, as we venture into the second leg, things will get a notch higher. We're talking about beefing up both your upper and lower body strength. Expect to meet poses and sequences that focus on working out your arms, shoulders, legs, and core. It's all about building that strength and resilience.

Days 11 to 15: The Whole Package

The final stretch of our journey is about bringing it all together in a full-body experience. We're not just sticking to dynamic movements here but also emphasizing the synergy between mind, body, and breath. It is where everything comes together in a beautiful balance.

Customization With Mudras

And here's the cherry on top: mudras. These symbolic hand gestures in yoga aren't just cool to do; they channel energy flow and stimulate brain reflexes. Each day of our program gives you a sturdy structure, but feel free to sprinkle in your personal touch with mudras that align with your goals and needs. Looking for peace of mind, better focus, or an energy kick? There's a mudra for that. This way, your yoga practice becomes a routine and a reflection of your journey.

So, remember, this 15-day program isn't just about stretching and bending; it's a journey of self-discovery on and off the chair. Approach each day with a sense of wonder, and watch as the transformation unfolds. Let's start this journey to explore, grow, and bloom.

15-Day Chair Yoga Training: Progress Monitoring Tools

Welcome to each new phase of your 15-day Chair Yoga journey! As you embark on every 5-day routine—Day 1, Day 6, and Day 11—you have a unique opportunity to track your progress and witness your growth. Our Standard Progress Monitoring Tool is designed to be your companion at the start of each phase.

Here's how you can make the most of it:

- **Day 1, Day 6, and Day 11:** On these days, you'll fill out the Standard Progress Monitoring Tool. It's a moment to pause, reflect, and set your benchmarks.
- **Assess and reflect:** At the beginning of each 5-day routine, take some time to evaluate your current state in key areas: flexibility, strength, mindfulness, and overall well-being. This assessment isn't just about numbers; it's about tuning into your body and mind, understanding where you are, and setting intentions for the days

ahead.
- **Chart your journey:** As you progress through each 5-day cycle, this tool will help you chart your journey, providing insights into how the practices are enhancing different aspects of your physical and mental health.
- **Celebrate your growth:** By tracking your progress at these intervals, you'll be able to see just how far you've come, celebrate your achievements, and identify areas for continued focus and improvement.

Let this tool guide your exploration and deepen your connection to the transformative power of chair yoga. Remember, each step forward, no matter how small is a part of your journey toward a healthier, more balanced self.

Ready to begin? Let's embrace this journey with heart and mindfulness, one breath, one pose, one day at a time

Flexibility & Mobility Journal

Description: Note down the specific stretches or poses you practiced.

Starting Feel: Rate your initial flexibility level on a scale of 1 (very stiff) to 10 (very flexible).

End Feel: Rate your flexibility level after the routine on the same scale.

Observations: Describe any improvements, areas of tension, or ease you felt in certain stretches.

Strength & Balance Tracker

Description: List the strength or balance poses you worked on.

Hold Duration: Note the duration you could hold the pose initially and after practicing.

Stability: Rate your stability on a scale of 1 (very unstable) to 10 (very stable).

Observations: Mention any improvements in holding times or increased stability in specific poses.

Mindfulness & Breathing Log

Description: Note the mindfulness practices or breathing exercises you engaged in.

Starting Calmness: Rate your initial state of mind on a scale of 1 (very restless) to 10 (very calm).

End calmness: Rate your state of mind after the practice on the same scale.

Observations: Describe any changes in your mental state, clarity, or relaxation levels.

General Wellbeing Feedback

Description: List any general exercises or routines you practiced.

Energy Levels: Rate your energy before and after the routine on a scale of 1 (very tired) to 10 (very energetic).

Mood: Describe your mood in a few words both before and after the practice.

Observations: Note any changes in overall well-being, mood upliftment, or general feelings post-practice.

Days 1 to 5: Laying Down the Foundations

FOCUS

This initial phase is dedicated to establishing a solid groundwork in chair yoga practice. The focus will be on mastering fundamental postures, honing balance, and enhancing flexibility. Participants will engage in simple yet effective exercises that emphasize proper posture and alignment. Breathing techniques will also be introduced to foster a deeper connection between mind and body, laying the foundation for a sustainable and safe yoga practice. This period is crucial for building confidence and understanding the basics, ensuring a strong and informed start to the journey.

1. **Mountain Pose Chair** (Please refer to the detailed description on page 54)
2. **Seated Shoulder Circles Chair** (Please refer to the detailed description on page 103)
3. **Pigeon Pose Chair** (Please refer to the detailed description on page 59)
4. **Cow Pose Chair** (Please refer to the detailed description on page 61)
5. **Goddess Pose On Chair** (Please refer to the detailed description on page 111)
6. **Easy Pose Chair One Leg Opposite Arm Raised** (New Pose)

Easy Pose Chair One Leg Opposite Arm Raised

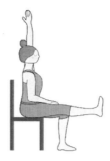

Easy Pose Chair One Leg Opposite Arm Raised is a seated yoga pose performed with one leg raised and the opposite arm extended. In this pose, you sit on a chair, maintaining balance and alignment while engaging various muscle groups.

Easy Pose Chair One Leg Opposite Arm Raised challenges your balance and concentration, helping improve your mind-body connection.

This pose engages the quadriceps and hip muscles, contributing to leg strength and stability.

It encourages flexibility in the raised leg and arm while enhancing the range of motion in the hip.

While this pose offers several benefits, individuals with certain conditions or limitations should exercise caution.

Should you have a recent or ongoing hip, knee, or ankle injury, it's advised to seek guidance from a healthcare expert or yoga teacher before attempting this pose.

Individuals with severe balance issues or vertigo may want to avoid this pose or practice it with a wall or chair back support.

Steps (3 minutes)

1. Sit comfortably on a chair with your feet firmly grounded on the floor.
2. Maintain an upright posture, with your spine straight and core engaged.
3. Inhale as you raise one leg, extending it parallel to the floor.
4. Simultaneously, lift the opposite arm, reaching it towards the ceiling or sky.
5. Find your balance in this position, focusing on stability and lengthening in the raised leg and arm. Hold this position for 3 minutes.

Breath Deeply and Let Go

Day 1 to Day 5: Building a Strong Foundation

Hands page 41
page 54

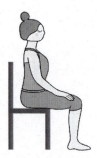

Mountain Pose Chair
(2 minutes)

Begin seated on a chair with feet flat. Close your eyes and breathe deeply for two breaths. Place the right hand on the belly and, the left on the chest, and focus on the breath for ten breaths for 2 minutes

Hands page 39
page 104

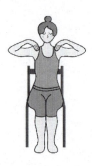

Seated Shoulder Circles Chair
(2 minutes)

Sit upright in the Mountain Pose Chair with fingertips touching the shoulders. Try to touch bent elbows in front. While inhaling, raise your arms, pointing elbows upward, then move them backward. On an exhale, lower the elbows to your sides and then bring them forward. Continue this motion for 1 minute, then relax. Reverse the direction for another 1 minute and conclude by resting your arms at your sides.

Page 60

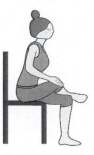

Pigeon Pose Chair
(2 minutes)

Gently, with an inhale, the right leg is lifted by the hands, gracefully crossing it over the left thigh. Ensuring comfort remains paramount in this position. As the leg finds its resting place, the practitioner is encouraged to straighten the spine, embracing the calm for 2 minutes. For those finding the leg cross challenging, a modified approach involves simply cradling the right leg before a slow release.

All pose images are copyright by Tummee - sequencing platform for yoga teachers

Hands page 37
page 62

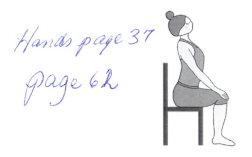

Cow Pose Chair
(3 minutes)
Sit on a chair with feet flat and hands on thighs. Inhale, arch your back, push your chest forward, and gently tilt your head back. Exhale and return to a neutral position. Repeat, moving with your breath, for 3 minutes.

Hands page 37
page 112

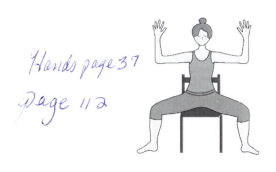

Goddess Pose On Chair
(3 minutes)
Spread your feet wider than your hips and angle your toes outward. With hands on your waist and a straight spine, inhale deeply, engaging your core. As you exhale, lean forward slightly. Align your knees with your ankles, grounding your feet firmly. Upon inhaling once more, stretch your arms into a cactus-like shape with your palms facing forward. Hold this position, gazing ahead with relaxed shoulders, for 3 minutes. Finally, exhale, return to the starting position, and relax, absorbing the benefits of the pose.

page 176

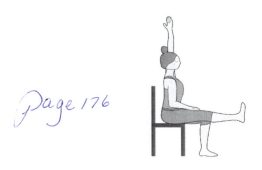

Easy Pose Chair One Leg Opposite Arm Raised
(3 minutes)
Sit comfortably on a chair with both feet planted firmly on the floor. Ensure an upright posture with a straight spine and engaged core muscles. As you inhale, lift one leg, extending it parallel to the floor. Simultaneously, raise the opposite arm towards the ceiling or sky. Maintain balance in this position for 3 minutes, emphasizing stability while elongating the raised leg and arm.

All pose images are copyright by Tummee - sequencing platform for yoga teachers

Tailored Checklist Routine for Days 15

As you journey through each day of your 5-day chair yoga routine, it's not just about performing the poses; it's about observing and understanding the progress you're making. To help you capture these subtle yet significant changes, we have developed a specialized progress monitoring tool tailored specifically for this segment of your yoga journey.

At the end of each day, after you have completed all six poses in the routine, take a moment to engage with this tool. It's designed to provide insightful feedback on key areas of your practice:

1. **Core Engagement Test:** This simple test will help you gauge the effectiveness of your core muscles. By measuring the gap under your lower back after a session, you can track improvements in core engagement over time.
2. **Posture self-assessment:** Awareness of your posture, both while sitting and standing, is crucial. This assessment allows you to reflect on your posture, noting any improvements or changes in alignment that have occurred as a result of your practice.
3. **Breath counts in core poses:** Counting your breaths while holding core-intensive poses is an excellent indicator of your stamina and core strength. Over time, an increase in breath count signifies progress in these areas.

This tailored progress monitoring is more than just a tracking tool; it's a reflective exercise that encourages you to connect deeply with your body's responses to the yoga practice. It helps in acknowledging the strides you're making, no matter how small, and in setting the stage for the next phase of your yoga journey. Remember, every little progress counts, and this tool is here to celebrate your journey towards better health and well-being.

Days 6 to 10: Boosting Strength in Upper and Lower Body

FOCUS

The focus for these days shifts to intensifying physical strength, particularly in the upper and lower body. Participants will be guided through a series of poses and movements that specifically target muscle groups in the arms, shoulders, legs, and core. This phase is designed to build upon the foundational flexibility and balance from the first phase, enhancing overall muscular strength and endurance. In addition to physical strengthening, there will be an emphasis on increasing mobility and agility, preparing the body for more dynamic and challenging sequences in the subsequent days.

1. **Neck Rolls Chair A-B-C** (Please refer to the detailed description on page 120)
2. **Seated Palm Tree Pose Side Bend Flow Chair** (New Pose)
3. **Torso Circles Chair** (New Pose)
4. **Seated Cactus Arms Chair** (Please refer to the detailed description on page 114)
5. **Flexing Foot Pose Chair** (Please refer to the detailed description on page 138)
6. **Wide-Legged Seated Twist Chair** (Please refer to the detailed description on page 143)

Seated Palm Tree Pose Side Bend Flow Chair

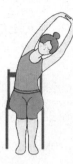

Seated Palm Tree Pose Side Bend Flow Chair involves a seated position on a chair with the arms raised and bent to the side. This pose primarily targets the muscles in the arms, shoulders, and upper back, and engages the biceps, triceps, and psoas muscles.

Practicing a Seated Palm Tree Pose Side Bend Flow Chair can help improve the strength and flexibility of the arms and shoulders. It offers a gentle stretch to the upper back, promoting better posture and spinal health. Additionally, this pose engages the biceps and triceps, aiding in toning and strengthening the arm muscles.

While enhancing the physical aspects, the Seated Palm Tree Pose Side Bend Flow Chair also encourages mental focus and concentration. The gentle flow and stretch of the pose can bring a sense of relaxation and mindfulness, making it suitable for stress relief and overall well-being.

There are no particular contraindications for the Seated Palm Tree Pose Side Bend Flow Chair, making it a suitable choice for a wide range of practitioners. However, as with any exercise, it's always wise to listen to your body and practice within your comfort zone.

Steps (2 minutes)

1. Start by sitting on a chair with your feet flat on the ground.
2. Ensure an upright posture, engage your core muscles, and release any shoulder tension.
3. Stretch both arms outward to the sides at shoulder level.
4. Inhale deeply, and as you exhale, bend one arm to the side, lowering your upper body toward that side.
5. Keep your opposite arm extended, creating a side bend.
6. Feel the stretch along the side of your body as you hold the position for 1 minute.
7. Inhale and return to the upright position with both arms extended.
8. Exhale and repeat the side bend on the opposite side, stretching in the other direction. Hold this position for 1 minute.
9. Continue to alternate between both sides, flowing with your breath.
10. Concentrate on the subtle stretch and the soothing flow of this movement.

Torso Circles Chair

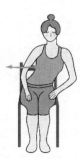

Torso Circles Chair is a gentle and supportive yoga practice performed while seated on a chair. It involves circular movements of the torso in both clockwise and counterclockwise directions, synchronized with your breath. This practice offers various physical and mental benefits.

Torso Circles Chair can be used as a warmup exercise before more intense yoga poses or flows.

Torso Circles Chair offers benefits to various muscle groups, including the hips, lower back, and middle back. This makes it a valuable addition to sequences focused on these areas.

Torso Circles Chair provides support for individuals recovering from conditions like Diastasis Recti or hip replacements.

For those with limited mobility or recovering from neck, back, and hip stiffness, this practice helps tone and strengthen muscles.

It's a great practice for individuals spending long hours at a desk, as it combats stiffness and keeps the spine active.

This practice has a calming effect on the body, promoting relaxation and activating the body's rest and digestion mechanism.

While Torso Circles Chair is generally safe, there are some precautions to consider. Individuals recovering from surgery or with specific medical conditions should practice it under the guidance of a medical professional or experienced yoga instructor. Care should also be taken with chair selection and the speed of movements.

In summary, Torso Circles Chair is a versatile yoga practice that offers support, relaxation, and flexibility benefits while being adaptable to various needs and conditions.

Steps (2 minutes)

1. Start by sitting up straight in a seated position.
2. Position your hands on your lower abdomen, with your palms resting on the sides of your belly.
3. Inhale as you initiate the Torso Circles Chair, moving from left to right.
4. While moving, observe how the abdominal side muscles engage, and press your palms gently into your sides.
5. Perform slow, rhythmic circles in a clockwise direction, and then repeat the movement in an anticlockwise direction.
6. Complete the movement for 2 minutes, 1 minute in each direction.
7. During exhalation, open your mouth and breathe out slowly, focusing on extending the exhalation and creating an audible sound.
8. As you exhale, consciously release tension in the spine and maintain a mindful and deliberate breathing pattern.

Day 6 to Day 10: Enhancing Upper and Lower Body Strength

Neck Rolls Chair A-B-C
(3 minutes)

Begin with Neck Roll A: lower your chin to your chest and then gently tilt your head back, repeating these forward and backward movements for 1 minute. For Neck Roll B, move your head side to side, bringing your ear towards each shoulder without raising the shoulders, alternating sides for 30 seconds each. Finish with Neck Roll C: turn your head to look over each shoulder, keeping your shoulders relaxed and facing forward, again for 30 seconds each side.

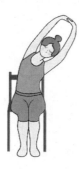

Seated Palm Tree Pose Side Bend Flow Chair
(2 minutes)

Sit up straight on a chair, engage your core, and relax your shoulders. Extend both arms to the sides at the level of your shoulders. As you inhale deeply, exhale and bend one arm to the side, lowering your upper body in that direction while keeping the opposite arm extended. Inhale again, returning to an upright position with both arms extended. Hold this position for 1 minute. Exhale and repeat the side bend on the opposite side, stretching in the opposite direction. Hold this position for 1 minute.

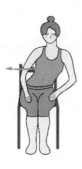

Torso Circles Chair
(2 minutes)

Begin seated with an upright posture, placing your hands on your lower abdomen. Inhale and initiate gentle circles, first clockwise and then anticlockwise, observing your abdominal muscles. Complete the movement for 2 minutes, 1 minute in each direction. During exhalation, breathe out audibly and mindfully, releasing tension in your spine.

All pose images are copyright by Tummee - sequencing platform for yoga teachers

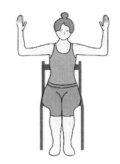

Seated Cactus Arms Chair
(3 minutes)

Sit upright with your feet flat, establishing a strong foundation. Inhale, lifting your arms to shoulder level, and as you exhale, bend your elbows into a cactus shape. Maintain this position. Deepen the pose for 3 minutes, expanding your chest and engaging your arm muscles. Return your arms to the center and then lower them to your knees. Conclude by relaxing and focusing on deep, rhythmic breathing.

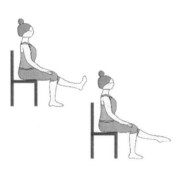

Flexing Foot Pose Chair
(2 minutes)

Seated on a chair, transition from a relaxed state to lifting one leg at a 40-degree angle. Flex the ankle and toes of the elevated leg up and down, repeating this about 1 minute. Feel the stretch in the Achilles tendon before switching to the other leg. Practice with caution, especially if inflammation is present.

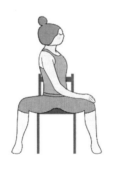

Wide-Legged Seated Twist Chair
(3 minutes)

Take a deep inhalation, seated on a chair with legs spread wide for balance. As you exhale, gently rotate your torso to the right, guiding the twist with your left hand on the right knee. After savoring the stretch across your spine and hips for 1 minute and a half, return to center on an inhalation. Repeat the twist towards the left, using your right hand for guidance. Conclude by settling back into a centered, relaxed position, letting the invigorating effects of the twist permeate your body.

Tailored Checklist Routine for Days 6 to 10

As you progress into the next phase of your 15-day chair yoga journey, spanning from Day 6 to Day 10, we focus more on enhancing your upper and lower body strength and your balance. To effectively track and understand your advancements in these areas, we have a specific set of progress monitoring tools tailored to this segment of your practice.

Each day, after completing your yoga routine, you will engage with this monitoring tool. It's a crucial part of your practice, helping you to recognize and appreciate the progress you're making in key areas of strength and balance:

1. **Seated heel-to-toe test:** This test is designed to assess balance in a safe, seated position. While sitting on a chair, extend one leg and place the heel of one foot directly in front of the toes of the other foot, creating a straight line. Try to maintain this heel-to-toe position for as long as possible without losing your balance or the alignment of your feet. Over time, an improvement in your ability to hold this position will indicate enhanced balance and coordination.

2. **Stability self-assessment:** After each session, take a moment to reflect on your feelings of stability, particularly during poses that involve one-legged stances or require balancing skills. Noting these feelings can help you gauge improvements or areas that need more focus.

3. **Chair stand test:** This exercise is designed to measure your leg strength and balance. Try to sit and stand from a chair without using your hands for support, and count the number of repetitions you can do in 30 seconds. An increase in repetitions over time signifies improved leg strength and overall balance.

This personalized approach to monitoring your progress is essential in understanding the effectiveness of your practice and in recognizing the strides you're making toward better health and well-being.

Days 11 to 15: The Whole Package

FOCUS

Focusing on integrating the body as a cohesive unit, this phase emphasizes the synchronization of movement, breath, and mindfulness. The routines are designed to harmonize upper and lower body strength with core stability, creating a seamless blend of physical agility and mental clarity. This stage aims to elevate the practice to a more holistic experience, ensuring that the benefits of chair yoga permeate both the physical and mental aspects of well-being.

1. **Mountain Pose Chair** (Please refer to the detailed description on page 54)

2. **Seated Forward Fold Pose Chair** (Pose Chair Please refer to the detailed description on page 82)

3. **Neck Rolls Chair A-B-C** (Please refer to the detailed description on page 120)

4. **Seated External Hip Rotation Pose Chair** (Please refer to the detailed description on page 146)

5. **Eagle Pose Chair** (New Pose)

6. **Seated Half Forward Fold Pose Chair Toes Forearms** (New Pose)

Eagle Pose Chair

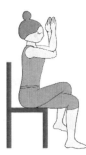

The Eagle Pose Chair is a versatile posture that targets various areas. In this pose, the arms and shoulders are actively engaged as one arm is crossed over the other, promoting strength and flexibility in these regions. Additionally, it offers a gentle but effective stretch to the upper back, which is particularly beneficial for alleviating tension and enhancing flexibility in this area. For the knees, the action of crossing the legs in this pose aids in improving joint mobility and providing a stretch.

However, the Eagle Pose Chair should be approached with care, especially for individuals with existing shoulder or arm injuries. In such cases, the pose should be modified or avoided to prevent discomfort. Similarly, those with significant knee issues are advised to seek guidance from a healthcare professional or yoga instructor before attempting this pose. Despite these considerations, the Eagle Pose Chair is a valuable addition to Chair Yoga sequences and can be adapted for a variety of practitioners, including those in prenatal or postnatal yoga.

Steps (2 minutes)

1. Start by sitting in a chair with your spine straight and your feet flat on the floor.
2. Inhale deeply while lifting your arms to shoulder height and extending them out to the sides.
3. Exhale and cross your right arm over your left arm, attempting to bring your palms together.
4. Bend your elbows to create an eagle arm bind, with your forearms perpendicular to the floor.
5. Inhale again and, on the exhale, cross your right thigh over your left thigh, tucking your right foot behind the left calf if possible.
6. Engage your core and maintain the pose for 1 minute.
7. To release, unravel your arms and legs, returning to the initial seated position.
8. Repeat the pose by switching sides, crossing the left arm over the right arm and the left thigh over the right thigh.
9. Hold the pose for an equal duration on both sides.

Seated Half Forward Fold Pose Chair Toes Forearms

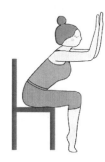

Seated Half Forward Fold Pose Chair Toes and Forearms involve specific benefits for various muscle groups.

This seated yoga pose on a chair targets the arms, shoulders, feet, ankles, hips, and psoas muscles. It is commonly included in Chair Yoga, prenatal yoga, and hip opening yoga sequences, offering benefits such as strengthening, flexibility, and hip opening. However, individuals with specific conditions should be cautious, and contraindications may apply in some cases.

While Seated Half Forward Fold Pose Chair Toes Forearms is generally a safe practice, it's important to be aware of potential contraindications, especially for individuals with specific conditions or considerations. Please consult with a yoga teacher or healthcare professional if you have concerns.

Steps (3 minutes)

1. Start by settling into a chair with your feet firmly on the ground and your knees bent at a right angle.
2. Stretch your spine upward, maintaining a straight back and an active core.
3. Lift your arms straight in front of you at shoulder height, and then raise your forearms to create a right angle with your arms.
4. Slowly bend forward from the hips, keeping your back straight.
5. Elevate your heels off the ground, pressing your toes firmly down as if you were trying to point at the ceiling with them.
6. Maintain this pose for 3 minutes, focusing on a long spine and the sensation of stretching in your back and the lower part of your legs.
7. To exit the pose, release your arms, straighten your back, and gently lower your heels back to the floor.

Every Step Is a Step Towards Tranquility

Day 11 to Day 15: Holistic Body Integration

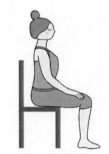

Mountain Pose Chair
(2 minutes)

Begin seated on a chair with feet flat. Close your eyes and breathe deeply for two breaths. Place the right hand on the belly and, the left on the chest, and focus on the breath for ten breaths for 2 minutes.

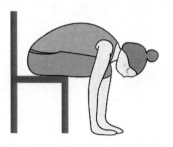

Seated Forward Fold Pose Chair
(3 minutes)

Starting in the Mountain Pose Chair (see p. 54), inhale and extend your torso. As you exhale, lower your arms towards your feet. Rest torso on thighs with chin near knees. Deepen the bend with each breath, aiming for palms on the floor. After holding for 3 minutes, return to the starting position.

Neck Rolls Chair A-B-C
(3 minutes)

Begin with Neck Roll A: lower your chin to your chest and then gently tilt your head back, repeating these forward and backward movements for 1 minute. For Neck Roll B, move your head side to side, bringing your ear towards each shoulder without raising the shoulders, alternating sides for 30 seconds each. Finish with Neck Roll C: turn your head to look over each shoulder, keeping your shoulders relaxed and facing forward, again for 30 seconds each side.

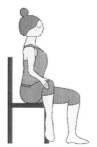

Seated External Hip Rotation Pose Chair
(2 minutes)

Seated on a comfortable chair with a straight spine and feet grounded. Lift one foot and place its ankle over the opposite knee in a figure four configuration. With the lifted foot flexed to ensure knee safety, the practitioner sits tall, feeling a gentle stretch in the hip. Hands rest gracefully on the lap or chair's armrests. Deep breaths enhance the stretch, providing relaxation. After 1 minute, the pose is repeated with the other leg, offering balanced flexibility.

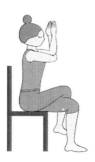

Eagle Pose Chair
(2 minutes)

In Eagle Pose Chair, start in a seated position on a chair with feet flat on the floor and spine erect. Inhale, raising arms to shoulder height, then exhale, crossing right arm over left, creating an eagle arm bind. Cross your right thigh over your left, and if possible, tuck your right foot behind your left calf. Engage the core, hold this position for 1 minute, and release, returning to the seated position. Repeat on the other side, holding for 1 minute.

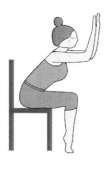

Seated Half Forward Fold Pose Chair Toes Forearms
(3 minutes)

Sitting comfortably in a chair, ground your feet and align your knees as you reach for a tall, straight spine. With your core engaged, extend your arms forward at shoulder height, then bend at the elbows to create right angles. As you lean forward from the hips, maintain the integrity of a straight back while lifting your heels, pressing your toes downward like you're reaching for the ceiling. Hold this stretch for 3 minutes, immersing in the elongation of your spine and the awakening of your legs' muscles.

Tailored Checklist Routine for Days 11 to 15

As you progress into the final phase of your 15-day Chair Yoga journey, it's time to reflect deeper on your holistic development. This tailored progress monitoring tool is designed to capture the essence of your growth in flexibility, fluidity of movements, and overall sense of well-being. By this stage, you're not only working on individual poses but also understanding how they seamlessly integrate to enhance your physical and mental harmony.

For each day, from Day 11 to Day 15, consider the following aspects:

- **Range in flexibility poses:** Focus on your flexibility range in various poses, particularly those that challenge your limits. Note specifics like how far your hands reach in a forward bend. Tracking this progress will highlight improvements in your physical flexibility over the days.
- **Integration feedback:** Pay attention to how smoothly you transition between poses. Smooth, effortless transitions are a sign of improved body integration and coordination. Jot down your observations about the fluidity and ease with which you move from one pose to another.
- **Holistic reflection:** At the end of each session, take a moment for introspection. Reflect on how the entire routine felt—did the poses flow more naturally? Did you notice increased body awareness? Write a few sentences about your overall feelings of well-being and any improvements in pose execution.

Remember, this tool is for assessing physical progress and acknowledging and celebrating the journey of your body and mind working in harmony. Embrace these final days with a spirit of exploration and self-discovery.

Conclusion

As we turn the final page of this particular passage in our chair yoga narrative, let's pause to appreciate the fullness of the expedition we've undertaken. It isn't merely the conclusion of a series of stretches and poses; it's the culmination of countless moments of self-discovery and personal triumph.

Chair Yoga: A Practice for a Lifetime

It isn't just a statement—it's a testament to the enduring power of gentle, intentional movement. Our journey together through this accessible form of yoga has woven a rich tapestry that illustrates the adaptability of the human spirit and the boundless capacity of our bodies for renewal and rejuvenation.

In our sessions, each seated sun salutation, each twist, and extension wasn't simply a physical act—it was an act of reclamation. We claimed moments of our day to care for our bodies, to honor our needs, and to engage with our breath. We found solace in the chair's stability and liberation in the movements that took us beyond its confines.

This practice has become a silent partner in our quest for well-being, a partner that asks for nothing but our presence and rewards us with immeasurable riches—strength, flexibility, balance, and peace of mind. With each stretch, we reach further into the possibilities of what our bodies can do, not defined by age or convention but by the courage to try and the will to continue.

The beauty of chair yoga lies in its simplicity and the profound effect it can have. It's a reminder that our physical limitations are not barriers but starting points from which we can explore our potential. It teaches us that our journey through life's seasons is not about the heights we ascend but about the depth of our roots and the breadth of our embrace.

In the quiet moments of reflection that follow our practice, we find a resonance that vibrates through the rest of our lives. The lessons of patience, moving with grace, breathing through challenges, and finding equilibrium translate into our daily interactions and our approach to life's unpredictable rhythms.

As you integrate chair yoga into the narrative of your daily life, let the chair be not just a piece of furniture but a foundation—a place from which you can reach, bend, twist, and expand. It is from this foundation that you will continue to grow, not just in your physical capabilities but in your capacity for joy, wonder, and contentment.

And so, as we conclude, remember that every ending is laced with the promise of a new beginning. Chair yoga has opened a door that never closes—a door to a practice that is as timeless as it is timely. It's a practice that you can return to repeatedly, each time with fresh eyes and an open heart.

Thank you for embarking on this chair yoga journey, for bringing your full self to the practice, and for embracing the myriad ways it can enrich your life. May you carry its essence with you, finding in each pose a reminder of your strength, in each breath a reminder of your resilience, and in each moment a reminder of your capacity for renewal.

Here's to the journey ahead, paved with the intentions and transformations that chair yoga has inspired. May it continue to be a source of strength, a moment of respite, and a beacon of joy in the ever-unfolding story of your life.

Glossary

Introduction

Welcome to the Glossary of Chair Yoga Poses! This section is designed as a quick reference guide to help you easily navigate through the various yoga poses featured in this book. Whether you're a seasoned practitioner or new to chair yoga, this glossary will be a handy tool to enrich your understanding and practice.

How to Use This Glossary

Pose Names: Each entry begins with the name of the yoga pose, presented in both English and Sanskrit (if applicable). This dual naming system will acquaint you with the traditional yoga terminology while keeping it accessible.

Visual Guide: Accompanying each pose name is a clear, illustrative image. These visuals provide a snapshot of the pose, aiding in recognition and understanding.

Page References: For each pose, you'll find two key page references:

Detailed Description: This page number leads you to the full description of the pose, where you can find step-by-step instructions.

Scheme Page: This page number directs you to the scheme page where the pose is included. The scheme pages offer a quick, visual summary of the pose sequences, ideal for practice sessions.

Feel free to use this glossary as a companion to your daily practice or as a reference guide to deepen your knowledge of chair yoga. It's here to help you seamlessly integrate the wisdom of yoga into your life, enhancing your journey towards health and well-being.

POSE / MUDRA NAME	IMAGE	TYPE	PAGE FOR DETAILED DESCRIPTION	SCHEME PAGE REFERENCE
Anjali Mudra		Mudra	33	44, 66, 80
Ankle Crank On Chair		Yoga Pose	157	168
Apana Mudra		Mudra	41	48, 66, 95, 134, 152, 169
Bicep Curl Exercise Chair		Yoga Pose	72	80
Bound Hands Chair		Yoga Pose	74	81
Cat Pose Variation		Yoga Pose	78	81
Cat Pose Variation Elbows		Yoga Pose	76	81
Cobra Pose Chair		Yoga Pose	90	95
Cobra Pose Chair Variation Hands Chest		Yoga Pose	92	95
Cow Pose Chair		Yoga Pose	61	67, 179
Dhyana Mudra		Mudra	40	46, 51, 67, 81, 134, 169
Eagle Pose Chair		Yoga Pose	191	197
Easy Pose Chair One Leg Raised		Yoga Pose	163	169
Easy Pose Chair One Leg Opposite Arm Raised		Yoga Pose	175	179
Flexing Foot Pose Chair		Yoga Pose	138	152, 187
Goddess Pose On Chair		Yoga Pose	111	119, 179
Goddess Pose with Arms Down		Yoga Pose	159	168
Half Seated Forward Bend Pose Chair		Yoga Pose	154	168

All pose images are copyright by Tummee - sequencing platform for yoga teachers

POSE / MUDRA NAME	IMAGE	TYPE	PAGE FOR DETAILED DESCRIPTION	SCHEME PAGE REFERENCE
Hands Chest Chair		Yoga Pose	55	66
Hands Up Chair		Yoga Pose	106	118
Head Up Chair		Yoga Pose	88	95
Jala Mudra		Mudra	42	49, 80, 95, 118, 153, 168
Kali Mudra		Mudra	34	49, 135
Knee Head Down Chair		Yoga Pose	161	169
Lotus Mudra		Mudra	38	46, 119, 135
Mountain Pose Chair		Yoga Pose	54	66, 178, 196
Mountain Pose Heel Raised Chair		Yoga Pose	63	67
Mountain Pose Raised Hands Chair		Yoga Pose	116	119
Mushti Mudra		Mudra	39	45, 50, 80, 94, 118, 134, 152, 168
Neck Rolls A Chair		Yoga Pose	120	134, 186, 196
Neck Rolls B Chair		Yoga Pose	120	134, 186, 196
Neck Rolls C Chair		Yoga Pose	120	134, 186, 196
Neck Stretch Chair		Yoga Pose	123	134
Pigeon Pose Chair		Yoga Pose	59	67, 178
Seated Cactus Arms Chair		Yoga Pose	114	119, 187
Seated Cactus Arms Together Chair		Yoga Pose	127	135
Seated External Hip Rotation Pose Chair		Yoga Pose	146	153, 197
Seated Forward Fold Pose Chair Variation Arm Crossed		Yoga Pose	86	94
Seated Forward Fold Pose Chair		Yoga Pose	82	94, 196
Seated Half Forward Fold Pose Chair		Yoga Pose	84	94

All pose images are copyright by Tummee - sequencing platform for yoga teachers

POSE / MUDRA NAME	IMAGE	TYPE	PAGE FOR DETAILED DESCRIPTION	SCHEME PAGE REFERENCE
Seated Half Forward Fold Pose Chair Toes Forearms		Yoga Pose	193	197
Seated Half Wind Release Pose I Chair		Yoga Pose	141	152
Seated Hip Circle Chair		Yoga Pose	165	169
Seated Palm Tree Pose Side Bend Flow Chair		Yoga Pose	182	186
Seated Pigeon Pose Arms Raised Chair		Yoga Pose	70	80
Sited Pigeon Pose Palms Up Chair		Yoga Pose	68	80
Seated Shoulder Circles Chair		Yoga Pose	103	118, 178
Seated Side Stretch Pose Chair		Yoga Pose	125	134
Seated Twists Chair		Yoga Pose	108	118
Seated Windshield Wiper Pose Chair		Yoga Pose	150	153
Seated With Eagle Arms On Chair		Yoga Pose	131	135
Staff Pose Chair II		Yoga Pose	148	153
Tattva Mudra		Mudra	35	67, 81, 94, 118, 135, 152, 169
Three-Part Breath Chair		Yoga Pose	57	66
Torso Circles Chair		Yoga Pose	184	186
Upward Hand Stretch Pose Chair		Yoga Pose	129	135
Vayu Mudra		Mudra	36	45, 66, 94, 119, 153
Vitarka Mudra		Mudra	37	67, 81, 95, 119, 153, 168
Wide-Legged Seated Twist Chair		Yoga Pose	143	152, 187

All pose images are copyright by Tummee - sequencing platform for yoga teachers

Dear Reader,

It is my pleasure to offer you an exclusive opportunity to enhance your journey toward wellness and serenity. As a token of gratitude, you will receive the following bonuses as a gift, designed to deepen your practice and enrich your life.

Balance and Grace: Core Training for the Golden Years

Strengthen your core and improve your balance with a series of chair yoga exercises specifically designed for the golden years. This detailed guide offers targeted exercises that support stability and grace in everyday movements, helping you maintain proper posture and prevent falls.

Healthy Recipes for Yoga Enthusiasts

Discover nourishing recipes that marry flavor with wellness, specifically crafted for the yoga lifestyle. Enjoy meals that feed both your body and soul, ensuring every bite supports your journey to health and harmony.

Tips for Creating a Relaxing Yoga Space at Home

Learn how to transform any corner of your home into a tranquil yoga retreat. This guide offers simple, effective strategies for designing a peaceful yoga environment, from color choices to layout, to enhance your daily practice.

Mindfulness and Meditation

Delve into the art of mindfulness with practical techniques to cultivate a peaceful, centered state of being. This guide is your companion in exploring meditation practices that bring clarity, peace, and balance to your life.

Yoga Breathing Techniques

Elevate your yoga practice and daily life with powerful breathing techniques. Gain insights into harnessing the power of your breath for enhanced mental clarity, physical vitality, and overall life balance.

Below you will find a QR CODE that will give you direct access to these bonuses. I hope you will appreciate it.

To communicate with me directly, (or if you have any problem with the download of extra content) please write to us at info@peggymitchellbooks.com

With warmest regards and best wishes.

THANK YOU

Thank you for embarking on the "Chair Yoga for Seniors" journey. We sincerely hope it enriches your life with vibrant health, joyful moments, and a sense of serene strength.

May this book bring you abundant positivity and good fortune in all your endeavors. If it has brightened your days, **please consider leaving a review**.

Use the QR CODE

Your thoughts and experiences are invaluable and deeply appreciated.